PREVENTION'S

SUPER
·FOODS·
COOKBOOK

250 Delicious Recipes
Using Nature's Healthiest Foods

By the Editors of **PREVENTION** Magazine
Compiled and edited by Jean Rogers, Food Editor,
PREVENTION Magazine Health Books

Rodale Press, Emmaus, Pennsylvania

Introduction by Joanne D'Agostino, author of *Italian Cooking for a Healthy Heart*
and *Convertible Cooking for a Healthy Heart*

Cover design by Stan Green
Cover photography by Angelo Caggiano

If you have any questions or comments concerning this book, please write:

Rodale Press
Book Readers' Service
33 East Minor Street
Emmaus, PA 18098

Library of Congress Cataloging-in-Publication Data

Prevention's super foods cookbook : 250 delicious recipes using nature's
    healthiest foods / by the editors of Prevention magazine ; compiled
and edited by Jean Rogers ; introduction by Joanne D'Agostino.
        p.   cm.
Abridged version of: The Healing foods cookbook. 1991.
Includes index.
    ISBN 0–87596–167–3   hardcover
    1. Nutrition.   2. Cookery (Natural foods)   I. Rogers, Jean.
II. Prevention (Emmaus, Pa.)   III. Healing foods cookbook.   IV. Title:
Super foods cookbook.
RA784.P738   1993
641.5'637—dc20   92–37485
                                              CIP

Distributed in the book trade by St. Martin's Press

2 4 6 8 10 9 7 5 3 1   hardcover

Notice: This book is intended as a reference volume only, not as a medical guide or manual for self-treatment. If you suspect that you have a medical problem, please seek competent medical care. Keep in mind that nutritional needs vary from person to person, depending upon age, sex, health status, and total diet. The foods discussed and recipes given here are designed to help you make informed decisions about your diet and health. They are not intended as a substitute for any treatment prescribed by your doctor.

Prevention's Super Foods Cookbook Staff:
  Editor: Jean Rogers
  Executive Editor: Debora Tkac
  Recipe Development: Rodale Food Center, Tom Ney, Director
  Home Economists, Rodale Food Center: JoAnn Brader,
  Anita Hirsch, M.S., R.D.
  Nutritional Consultant: Joanne D'Agostino, R.N.
  Art Director: Jane Knutila
  Designer: Lisa Gatti
  Photographer: Angelo Caggiano
  Photo Editor: Barbara Fritz
  Food Stylist: Anne Disrude
  Research Chief: Ann Yermish
  Senior Research Associate: Karen Lombardi Ingle
  Production Editor: Jane Sherman
  Copy Editor: Laura Stevens
  Editor in Chief: William Gottlieb
  Editor, *Prevention* Magazine: Mark Bricklin

Contents

Introduction

I'm sure you're aware of the pitfalls in the typical American diet. There's too much fat, too much cholesterol, too many calories, too much sodium, too little fiber, not enough nutrients. And these dietary excesses and shortcomings can lead to serious health problems, including heart disease, obesity, high blood pressure, and even many types of cancer.

One of the best ways to take charge of your health is by eating foods that deliver maximum amounts of good-for-you nutrients and minimum quantities of nasty dietary no-no's. But you may worry that such a super-healthy eating plan will seem too much like, well, a "diet," leaving you hungry and hankering for your old favorite foods. You needn't fret! I can assure you that light, lean, and super-nutritious *can* be synonymous with great-tasting, satisfying, and indulgent.

My family and I have been enjoying low-fat, nutrient-rich meals for over five years. And we've never looked back, never missed the foods we "can't eat." Because truthfully, there's very little we can't have. We still relish our heirloom Italian recipes, still savor creamy cheesecakes and other desserts, still treat guests to the kinds of foods they love—without compromising our commitment to a healthy lifestyle. And you can, too.

We've learned how to cut fat and cholesterol without sacrificing flavor. How to remove salt and still get great taste. How to trim calories and yet finish dinner feeling full and satisfied. We've tapped into the secrets inherent in "super foods"—nutrient-packed foods as varied and delicious as meat, cheese, and seafood. As luscious as juicy ripe berries, peaches, and melons. As appealing as vibrant red, green, and orange vegetables. As filling as potatoes, pasta, and wonderful new grains.

You, too, can reap the benefits of super foods. The 250 delicious, low-fat, high-health recipes in *Prevention's Super Foods Cookbook* can show you how it's done and get you started on the road to good health. Let them be your ticket to a life where *diet* is no longer a four-letter word and where you *can* get satisfaction at every meal.

Joanne D'Agostino

Joanne D'Agostino
Author of *Italian Cooking for a Healthy Heart*
and *Convertible Cooking for a Healthy Heart*

CHAPTER ONE ◇

Foods for Super Health

The cornerstone of good health is a good diet—one packed with foods offering essential health-giving vitamins and minerals without being laden with fat and calories. And that's what the super foods highlighted in this chapter have to offer.

You won't be surprised to find that a lot of these foods are vegetables and fruits. That's because produce, perhaps more than any other foods, offers a wide variety of vitamins and minerals but no cholesterol, almost no fat or sodium, and very few calories.

Broccoli, for instance, is a nutrient giant. It's low in calories to help promote weight loss. But there's more: As a cruciferous vegetable, it may decrease the risk of certain cancers. As a high-fiber, high-potassium, low-sodium food, it helps combat heart disease and high blood pressure. And as a good source of calcium, it can help guard against osteoporosis. Other produce is equally impressive. Carrots, cabbages, apples, pumpkins, potatoes, winter squash, and other fresh foods earned their places on our list by being outstanding sources of health-building nutrients.

Some of the other foods may surprise you. Beef, pork, and lamb, for example, have a reputation as dietary no-no's. But all are good sources of iron and can be part of a healthy diet if you choose lean cuts and use them in moderation. And you may wonder if celery and mushrooms, for instance, have enough nutrients to qualify as super foods. The answer is that their strong point is exceptional *flavor*—enough to perk up a low-fat, low-salt diet so that you can stay with it and reap its healthy benefits.

Certain foods on this list may be unfamiliar to you, but they're worth getting to know. For example, papayas, mangoes, and other tropical fruits have more than sun-drenched flavor; they're high in fiber and vitamins A and C. Quinoa, an unusual grain, is loaded with protein to help supplement a reduced-meat diet. Other oft-neglected grains such as buckwheat, bulgur, and millet can add a new dimension to your diet.

All of which brings up an important point: A *varied* diet supplies a wide range of nutrients and keeps you from falling into a culinary rut. So variety is also what the list is all about.

If you make the foods in this chapter an integral part of your diet, you'll be using nature's best to safeguard your health. But keep in mind that a lifetime habit of healthy eating begins with meals that you truly enjoy. So use these super foods and the recipes that follow to enrich your diet and your well-being.

◇　　　◇　　　◇

Apples: One a day will do it. Just one

apple delivers 4.3 grams of dietary fiber—about as much as two slices of whole wheat bread. Most of it is in the insoluble form that prevents constipation. The rest is pectin, which studies have shown can lower cholesterol levels. Apples are also low in sodium, calories, and fat. And they're a great source of boron, which may help prevent the calcium losses that can lead to osteoporosis.

◇　　　◇　　　◇

Apricots: Brimming with beta-carotene. These sweet-tart treats are packed with

fiber and beta-carotene, the plant form of vitamin A that may have anticancer activity. Fresh apricots are practically calorie-free, containing only about 17 calories. Dried apricots have more calories, but ½ cup still contains only about 150. In addition,

apricots are high in potassium and low in sodium—a combination that is beneficial for preventing or controlling high blood pressure.

◇　　　◇　　　◇

Artichokes: Dip into fiber. This

unusual vegetable contains amazing amounts of fiber, with one medium artichoke weighing in with 5.2 grams. That's more than you get in a whole bowl of oat-bran cereal. And that gives you a good head start on the 20 to 30 grams of fiber a day the National Cancer Institute recommends for optimum health. Weight watchers should note that a whole medium 'choke has a mere 53 calories (as long as you forgo the hollandaise sauce). Besides that, eating an artichoke properly takes *time,* which can help overeaters control their appetites.

◇　　　◇　　　◇

Asparagus: Nutritional star of spring. These elegant spears are a dieter's dream—

12 large spears have only 45 calories. Those same stalks contain about 30 percent of the Recommended Dietary Allowance (RDA) for vitamin A and a generous amount of potassium. Like other vegetables, asparagus contains no cholesterol and virtually no fat, making it a boon for those concerned about heart health.

◇　　　◇　　　◇

Avocados: Rich in more ways than one. Here's one rich, buttery food that's good for

you. That's because it contains lots of monoun-saturated fat, which can actually help lower cholesterol. Additionally, avocados are awesome sources of potassium and very low in sodium, for double protection against high blood pressure. The avocado's only drawback: high calories and fat for a fruit. So be sure to cut back calories and fat elsewhere in your diet to compensate.

◇   ◇   ◇

Bananas: *An appealing fruit.*

A creamy-textured, medium banana has only 105 calories and the barest trace of fat. But it's got lots of potassium—so much that physicians often prescribe bananas as part of a regimen to help lower blood pressure.

◇   ◇   ◇

Barley: *Down with cholesterol.*

This healthy, high-fiber grain has lots of cholesterol-lowering potential. In one study, volunteers who ate barley fiber daily lowered both their total cholesterol and their harmful LDL cholesterol. In addition, barley's high in fiber and low in sodium. The two most common forms are Scotch and pearled. Scotch retains the bran and therefore has more fiber; soak it overnight before cooking.

◇   ◇   ◇

Beans: *Powerful protectors.*

These health champs are an excellent source of complex carbohydrates, protein, iron, and calcium. But their prime claim to fame is their soluble fiber: Cholesterol researcher James W. Anderson, M.D., advocates a diet high in dried beans for cholesterol control. And beans are terrific for weight watchers. One study showed beans can suppress the appetite for hours because they are digested very slowly. With about 125 calories per ½ cup, cooked beans are a lean choice. Fresh beans—snap, wax, Italian, and others—share most of the attributes of dried beans. But since they're not as dense, they are lower in fiber and certain nutrients. Still, they have lots of vitamins A and C, nutrients that dried beans lack. And ½ cup has just 22 calories.

◇   ◇   ◇

Beef: *Keep it lean.*

The key to healthy meat eating is to choose lean cuts such as flank steak and skirt steak. Then trim all visible fat before cooking. When working with ground beef, buy the leanest available and microwave it. Super-lean ground beef retains less fat when it is microwaved on paper towels than when it is roasted, broiled, or pan-fried. Beef packs a concentrated dose of vitamins and minerals. A 3-ounce serving of cooked lean beef contains about 17 percent of a woman's daily requirement for blood-building iron, and it's a very good source of zinc and B vitamins.

◇   ◇   ◇

Beets: *Unbeatable vegetables.*

One whole cup of cooked sliced beets has only 52 calories and no fat. That same cup has 3.4 grams of fiber, equal to 1½ cups of oatmeal. Remember that you can eat beets raw—and they have twice as much vitamin C as cooked ones. So shred some into salads for a crunchy taste treat. For variety, seek out yellow beets.

◇   ◇   ◇

Berries: *Diet delights.*

Take your choice—blueberries, raspberries, strawberries, blackberries, and more. All are low in calories, high in fiber, and great sources of vitamin C and potassium. And they're tailor-made for snacks and healthy desserts. Don't forget cranberries: Although they need sweetening, you can pair them with apples, oranges, or dried apricots instead of sugar.

(The raw berries also contain vitamin C, so use them in uncooked cranberry sauce.)

◇ ◇ ◇

Bran: **Full of fiber.** All types of bran are wonderful sources of both insoluble and soluble fiber. Insoluble fiber, the kind prominent in wheat bran, helps relieve constipation and may prevent hemorrhoids as well as diverticular disease. Soluble fiber—found in outstanding quantities in oat, corn, and rice brans—can help lower cholesterol. Although oat bran has gotten the most notice, the others are tasty additions to a health-building diet.

◇ ◇ ◇

Broccoli: **Stalk trouble before it strikes.** Broccoli is a member of the crucifer family of vegetables, and studies have suggested that a diet rich in these veggies may decrease cancer risks. Broccoli is also packed with beta-carotene, vitamin C, fiber, and potassium. And it even contains bone-building calcium. At least one study suggests that you can get the most benefit from broccoli by eating it raw, so cover all bases by enjoying it both cooked and au naturel.

◇ ◇ ◇

Brussels sprouts: **Little packages of potassium.** These little cabbages are also crucifers. Although they have considerably less calcium than broccoli when cooked, the two are on par when raw. Cooked sprouts have as much vitamin C and iron as broccoli and almost twice as much potassium. A tip: If you think you don't like brussels sprouts, try cooking them until *just* tender.

Overcooking produces the strong flavor many people dislike.

◇ ◇ ◇

Buckwheat: **Flour power—and kasha, too.** Buckwheat is actually an herb whose seeds are either eaten whole as groats or ground into flour. Unlike grains such as wheat and rye, buckwheat has no gluten, so it's suitable for people with gluten allergies. Buckwheat is low in fat and calories—½ cup of cooked groats (kasha) contains 97 calories—and high in fiber and protein. And it's digested very slowly, which may help curb your appetite. Many recipes call for coating the groats with beaten egg before cooking. If you're cutting cholesterol, use egg whites or egg substitute.

◇ ◇ ◇

Bulgur: **A quick fiber option.** Bulgur is a whole-grain product made from wheat kernels that have been steamed, dried, and crushed. This process lets you prepare bulgur very quickly as a substitute for long-cooking brown rice. Because only a small part of the bran is lost during processing, bulgur is nutritionally almost identical to whole wheat. That means it contains dietary fiber as well as B vitamins and iron.

◇ ◇ ◇

Cabbage: **King of the crucifers.** This wonderful vegetable comes in so many varieties that you'll never tire of it. And that's good, because crucifers in general may reduce the risk of gastrointestinal and respiratory-tract cancers. Because crucifers may work their wonders best when raw, try to include lots of uncooked cabbage in your diet. Dieters, take note: ½ cup of shredded cabbage contains a minuscule 8 calories.

◇   ◇   ◇

Carrots: *vitamin A plus.* Carrots are

chock-full with beta-carotene. Further, researchers say that just adding two carrots a day to your diet can reduce cholesterol by as much as 20 percent, which can help lessen the threat of heart disease. And if you substitute crunchy, chewy carrots for less-nutritious snacks, your weight may go down—a whole large carrot has just 31 calories.

◇   ◇   ◇

Cauliflower: *Ahead in health.* A

tasty ½ cup of cooked florets has just 15 calories plus lots of potassium and a bare trace of sodium. The same ½ cup contains about 50 percent of the RDA for vitamin C to help build immunity and increase iron absorption. And cauliflower is another cancer-fighting cruciferous vegetable. (What's more, scientists are in the process of breeding a bright orange variety that would taste the same but pack 100 times more cancer-blocking carotene.)

◇   ◇   ◇

Celery: *Versatile flavor enhancer.*

This dieter's favorite isn't all that high in nutrients, but it delivers big flavor for few calories and no fat. And it's so versatile that it can accent just about any dish. Celery does contain some sodium, but that taste of salt may be just enough to keep you from reaching for the saltshaker. And celery has lots of potassium to help prevent high blood pressure.

◇   ◇   ◇

Cheese: *Say calcium, please.* Low-

fat cheese fits into a heart-healthy diet. A 1-ounce slice provides protein, calcium, and only a modest amount of calories. As the chart on page 6 shows, some cheeses that are lowest in fat include Sapsago (a hard skim-milk product from Switzerland), pot cheese (a drier form of cottage cheese), and yogurt cheese. Interesting news: Cheese contains tryptophan, an amino acid that helps the brain regulate sleep. And cheese may even benefit your teeth by re-mineralizing them and also by reducing acids that cause plaque and lead to cavities.

◇   ◇   ◇

Chestnuts: *Autumn's slim pickings.*

These dark-shelled beauties are by far the slimmest nuts. A large handful has about 175 calories and less than 2 grams of fat. And that fat is largely the beneficial unsaturated type. Chestnuts also contain pectin, a water-soluble fiber that may help curb overeating because it slows the digestive process. And shelling chestnuts one by one as you nibble certainly slows the *eating* process.

◇   ◇   ◇

Citrus fruits: *The secret's in the fiber.* Whether you choose oranges, grapefruit,

tangerines, or one of the many other types, citrus fruits are low in calories, fat, and sodium but high in potassium. The deep-colored varieties also contain cancer-preventing beta-carotene. But the big news is all the cholesterol-lowering pectin found in citrus fruits. And a few studies have noted that when vitamin C—so plentiful in citrus—is added to a pectin-rich diet, cholesterol levels drop even lower. Weight watchers have long used lemons and limes

PUT THESE CHEESES
ON YOUR MENUS

Cheese can be part of any healthy diet, as long as you select those that are lowest in fat and calories. Sapsago, for example, is virtually fat-free, so you can use it liberally in your recipes. In fact, you'll find it in many of the recipes in this book. (If it's not available in your area, Parmesan is an acceptable substitute.) You will still need to practice a little discretion when it comes to those cheeses higher in calories—such as Cheddar, Colby, and Muenster—especially if weight loss is your goal. Generally, though, if you limit your selection to the cheeses listed in this table, you can consider yourself on the right side of health.

Cheese	Serving	Fat (g)	Calories
Yogurt cheese, nonfat	1 oz.	0	17
Pot cheese	1 oz.	0	25
Gammelost	1 oz.	0.1–0.3	52–60
Sapsago	1 Tbsp.	0.4	12
Fromage blanc	1 oz.	0.5	18
Yogurt cheese, low-fat	1 oz.	0.6	30
Parmesan, grated	1 Tbsp.	1.9	29
Monterey Jack, processed	1 oz.	2.0	50
Cheddar, processed	1 oz.	2.0–4.0	50–70
Swiss, processed	1 oz.	2.0–4.0	50–70
Muenster, processed	1 oz.	2.0–5.0	50–85
Swiss, lite	1 oz.	2.0–6.0	50–97
Cheddar, lite	1 oz.	3.0–6.0	65–90
Edam, reduced-fat	1 oz.	3.1	65
String, lite	1 oz.	4.0–6.0	70–90
Mozzarella, part-skim	1 oz.	4.5	72
Scamorza, part-skim	1 oz.	5.0	70
Colby, low-fat	1 oz.	5.0	85
Muenster, lite	1 oz.	5.0	85
Farmer's	1 oz.	5.0–7.0	80–90
Feta	1 oz.	6.0	75
Monterey Jack, lite	1 oz.	6.0	80
Mozzarella, whole-milk	1 oz.	6.1	80
Neufchâtel	1 oz.	6.6	74

in lieu of butter and fatty dressings to perk up the taste of seafood, salads, and vegetables. And the tart juice even compensates for missing salt, so it can aid those on low-sodium diets.

◇　　　◇　　　◇

Corn: Kernels of health. Corn contains lots of fiber but little calories, fat, or sodium. And it contributes B vitamins, vitamin C, and potassium to a healthy diet. Corn contains no gluten, so both fresh kernels and dried products such as cornmeal, grits, and corn bran are suitable for those with gluten allergies. Although corn's not rich in vitamin A, yellow corn does contain some.

◇　　　◇　　　◇

Cottage cheese: More than diet food. A large part of low-fat cottage cheese's value is its ability to replace sour cream, cream cheese, and cheese spreads in many recipes—just blenderize it until smooth. Further, cottage cheese is so low in fat, calories, and cholesterol that it warrants a place in the diets of both weight watchers and those hoping to avoid heart disease. And its high-quality protein is a boon to vegetarians. The chart on page 8 shows how the different forms of cheese-curd products compare.

◇　　　◇　　　◇

Crustaceans: Vitamin sea. These shellfish go by other names: crab, shrimp, crayfish, and lobster. They're nicely low in calories—as long as you avoid the melted butter and tartar sauce. Three ounces of cooked king crab has only 82 calories. Blue crab, shrimp, and lobster are about the same, and crayfish are just slightly higher. Years ago, shellfish were thought to be high in cholesterol. Today we know that the amount is far less than originally believed. What's more important is their low amount of saturated fat, which plays a larger role than dietary cholesterol in the development of heart disease. Do note that some crustaceans are high in natural sodium.

◇　　　◇　　　◇

Cucumbers: Nothing but goodness. Cukes are valued more for what's *not* in them: fat, sodium, cholesterol, and calories (an entire ½ cup has only 7 calories). Just make sure to enjoy these vegetables fresh. Pickling adds a lot of sodium.

◇　　　◇　　　◇

Eggplant: Mediterranean "medicine." This deep purple vegetable is very low in calories, sodium, and fat but high in fiber. And some studies have suggested that some component of eggplant can actually help lower cholesterol. A warning: Eggplant soaks up fat like a sponge. So if you're sautéing it, use healthy monounsaturated oils such as olive and canola, and keep quantities down.

◇　　　◇　　　◇

Figs: First fruit of fiber. Five of these dried fruits contain an impressive 8.7 grams of dietary fiber. That's more than you'd get in three bran muffins. Part of the fiber is insoluble, which combats constipation. The rest is soluble to help lower cholesterol. Figs are also a respectable source of minerals, including iron, potassium, and zinc. For a taste treat, fill up on fresh figs. One medium fruit has only 37 calories.

◇　　　◇　　　◇

WHERE'S THE FAT?

Various types of cottage cheese and ricotta cheese may look alike, but they differ quite a bit in calories, cholesterol, and fat, including the percentage of calories that come from fat. Make it a point to use the lowest-fat product that satisfies your taste and desire for creaminess. All figures are for ½ cup.

Cheese	Calories	Fat (g)	Calories from Fat (%)	Cholesterol (mg)
Cottage, dry-curd	62	0.3	4	5
Cottage, 1% fat	82	1.2	13	5
Cottage, 2% fat	102	2.2	19	10
Cottage, creamed	109	4.7	39	16
Ricotta, part-skim	171	9.8	52	38
Ricotta, whole-milk	216	16.1	67	63

Fish: Striking nutritional oil. All fish contain omega-3 fatty acids, special fats that can keep your heart healthy by lowering cholesterol. The top sources of omega-3's are the fattier fish such as mackerel, herring, sablefish, bluefin tuna, and salmon. (Note that canning does not deplete omega-3's. And if you eat canned fish that has bones—such as sardines, salmon, and mackerel—you get a bonus of calcium.) Lower-fat fish such as cod, haddock, flounder, and mahimahi contain fewer omega-3's, but they are still a very lean, low-calorie alternative to red meat. So try to eat some type of fish at least twice a week. (See the chart on the opposite page for details.)

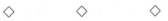

Game: Beef lover's alternative. Most game is lower in fat than regular red meat. And their fat is mostly polyunsaturated. A 3½-ounce serving of moose contains a mere 1.5 grams of fat; deer, 4 grams; and pheasant, 5.2. By comparison, the same portion of sirloin steak has 26.7 grams. Domestic rabbit is even lower in cholesterol than

FISHING FOR THE BEST

If you'd like to get a maximum benefit per mouthful, pay heed to this fish chart. It lists the best sources of omega-3's, those beneficial fats that may help reduce the risk of blood clots that could lead to heart attacks or strokes. Although the jury is still out on just how much of the omega-3's you need for good health, many doctors believe that as few as two to four fish meals a week may help. All figures are for 3½ ounces of uncooked seafood.

Seafood	Omega-3's (g)
Atlantic mackerel	2.6
Anchovies (canned)*	2.1
Atlantic herring	1.7
Atlantic salmon	1.7
Pink salmon (canned)	1.7
Sablefish	1.5
Chinook salmon	1.4
Whitefish	1.4
Sockeye salmon	1.3
Bluefin tuna	1.2
Coho salmon	1.0
Pink salmon	1.0

*Because of their high salt content, anchovies should not be eaten by those on a sodium-restricted diet.

chicken. Other pluses: Buffalo offers more protein and less fat and cholesterol than beef. Texas antelope gets only 5 percent of its calories from fat. And pheasant is both lean and very mild in taste.

◇   ◇   ◇

Garlic: *Keep heart disease at bay.*

Scientists are seriously examining the potential of garlic to protect against heart disease. Studies have shown that garlic raises beneficial HDL cholesterol while lowering total cholesterol. Garlic also thins the blood, reducing the chance of clotting. (Blood clots are a common cause of heart attack and stroke.) And a study from China suggests that allium vegetables, which include garlic and onions, may reduce the risk of stomach cancer.

◇   ◇   ◇

Grapes: *Divine eating.* These sweet

little jewels are low in calories—114 in a cupful.

And they have vitamins A and C, plus potassium. Grapes also contain boron, a mineral that could help safeguard calcium and thereby help prevent osteoporosis.

◇   ◇   ◇

Herbs and spices: Kick the salt habit.
Herbs and spices do contain some health-building vitamins and minerals, but most people don't eat them in large-enough quantity for those nutrients to be significant. The real benefit of these aromatics is their ability to perk up low-fat, low-sodium diets. No wonder these flavor enhancers are called the spice of life!

◇   ◇   ◇

Kale: Carotene and calcium.
This leafy green is another crucifer. It's rich in vitamins A and C, potassium, and fiber. One cup of raw leaves has more than a day's requirement of both A and C but just 33 calories. And kale is a good source of calcium. One cup of cooked frozen kale has 179 milligrams—as much as is in 1 ounce of mozzarella.

◇   ◇   ◇

Kiwifruit: Key in vitamin C.
Kiwi is low in calories—only 55 in a large fruit. And it's a great source of vitamin C, potassium, and fiber.

◇   ◇   ◇

Lamb: Link to iron and zinc.
Extra-lean lamb is loaded with iron to help prevent anemia. And it fits right into a healthy diet. A broiled, well-trimmed loin chop has just 92 calories and 3.7 grams of fat. That's not significantly more than a serving of dark-meat turkey. In addition,

lamb is a good source of zinc, and it's often an acceptable meat for those with food allergies.

◇   ◇   ◇

Mangoes: The color of carotene.
One cup of juicy mango slices has a modest amount of calories but lots of beta-carotene, vitamin C, fiber, and potassium. Mango even contains vitamin E, which some studies have linked to a reduced overall risk of cancer.

◇   ◇   ◇

Melons: Variety and vitamins.
Although the many varieties of melons may differ in taste and color, they're all low in calories, fat, and sodium. Melons also have valuable fiber, potassium, and vitamin C. As a bonus, the orange varieties such as cantaloupe contain cancer-fighting beta-carotene. Even watermelon has enough vitamin A to make it a valuable addition to your diet.

◇   ◇   ◇

Milk: Big benefits for bones.
Low-fat milk is our single best source of calcium, needed for strong bones. One cup of skim milk provides 38 percent of the RDA of 800 milligrams. (See the chart on the opposite page.) Milk is also a good source of B vitamins, especially B_{12}, as well as vitamin A and potassium. In addition, virtually all milk is enriched with vitamin D, which enhances calcium absorption. Research has shown that drinking low-fat milk may help lower total cholesterol levels.

◇   ◇   ◇

Millet: Easy on allergies.
This grain, which contains good amounts of B vitamins, iron, and potassium, tends to be tolerated well by people

IS YOUR MILK TOO FAT?

Here's how *your* favorite milk stacks up against the competition in terms of calories, fat, percentage of calories from fat, and milligrams of calcium. Don't be fooled by ads saying whole milk is only 4 percent fat. That's figured on a weight basis. The number of calories that come from fat—a more accurate assessment of health value—is considerably higher, tipping the scales at 49 percent. All figures below are for 1 cup of liquid milk.

Milk	Calories	Fat (g)	Calories from Fat (%)	Calcium (mg)
Evaporated skim, undiluted	198	0.5	2	738
Nonfat dry, reconstituted	81	0.2	2	279
Skim	86	0.4	5	302
Buttermilk	99	2.2	20	285
Low-fat (1%)	102	2.6	23	300
Low-fat (1%) with added calcium	102	3.0	26	500
Low-fat (2%)	121	4.7	35	297
Whole	150	8.2	49	291
Evaporated whole, undiluted	338	19.1	51	658

allergic to wheat or other grains. And it has protein that equals or exceeds that of rice, corn, and oats. With about 90 calories and very little fat per cooked cup, it's perfect for dieters. Like other whole grains, it has a decent amount of fiber for digestive health.

◇   ◇   ◇

Mollusks: **Minerals galore.** Oysters, clams, scallops, mussels, and other mollusks are much lower in cholesterol than once believed. And they contain virtually no saturated fat, making them a better dietary choice than even the leanest red meats. And mollusks have heart-healthy omega-3's, with mussels and oysters containing more than scallops and clams. In addition, clams, mussels, and oysters are high in iron. Oysters also contain plenty of zinc and a fair share of copper, which helps to regulate cholesterol metabolism.

◇   ◇   ◇

FAT IN A NUTSHELL

Here's how the most popular nuts rank in terms of monounsaturated fat. Macadamia nuts, those Hawaiian delicacies, lead the pack with 79 percent of their fat coming from beneficial monos. All values are for 1 ounce of nuts.

Nuts	Monounsaturated Fat (%)
Macadamia nuts	79
Hazelnuts, unblanched	78
Pistachio nuts	68
Almonds, unblanched	65
Pecans	62
Cashew nuts	59
Peanuts	50
Pine nuts	38
Brazil nuts, unblanched	35
English walnuts	23
Black walnuts	22

Mushrooms: **Weight-loss champignons.** These little morsels are ridiculously low in calories, with ½ cup of raw pieces having just 9 (½ cup cooked has just 21). And many varieties, such as shiitake, enoki, and porcini, have a meaty taste and texture, so they can help replace meat in many dishes. Like other vegetables, mushrooms are very high in potassium and low in sodium, the perfect formula for controlling high blood pressure.

◇   ◇   ◇

Nectarines: **Nutritiously well rounded.** Like its cousin the peach, the nectarine is low in calories yet well supplied with fiber and potassium. And it's a nice source of vitamins A and C.

◇   ◇   ◇

Nuts: **Mind your monos.** Many nuts are high in healthy monounsaturated fats, which have been shown to help lower cholesterol. (See the chart above.) Nuts are high in fiber and contain decent amounts of various minerals, including potassium. They're also quite low in sodium, as long as they're unsalted. Some—cashews and almonds in particular—are high in zinc. Further, nuts contain vitamin E, which may delay the onset of atherosclerosis. Their only drawback is their high fat and calorie count. So eat them in place of other fatty foods, not in addition to them.

◇   ◇   ◇

Oats: **Workhorse for the heart.** Although not as great a source of soluble fiber as oat

CHECK YOUR OIL

How does your favorite oil stack up in health value? Oils with the most cholesterol-lowering monounsaturates should make regular appearances on your table. And remember that even the best oils are a mixture of mono-unsaturated, polyunsaturated, and saturated fats. So use them judiciously.

Oil	Mono-unsaturated Fats (%)	Poly-unsaturated Fats (%)
Hazelnut	78	10
Olive	74	8
Almond	70	17
Avocado	70	16
Apricot kernel	60	29
Canola (rapeseed)	56	33
Peanut	46	32
Sesame	40	42
Rice bran	39	35
Corn	24	59
Soybean	23	58
Walnut	23	63
Linseed	20	66
Sunflower	20	66
Grapeseed	16	70
Wheat germ	15	62
Safflower	12	75

bran, rolled oats can still help reduce cholesterol in people with high levels of blood fat. Some doctors recommend aiming for at least 10 grams of fiber from oat products a day—a single serving of oatmeal gives you almost 3 grams. In addition to only 110 calories and hardly any fat per serving, oats contain potassium, B vitamins, and iron.

Oil: Olive and company strike it rich.

Most oils are composed largely of beneficial mono-unsaturated or polyunsaturated fats. Monos—found in olive, canola, rice-bran, and other oils (see the chart above)—can help lower total cholesterol and bad-for-you LDL cholesterol without reducing protective HDLs. Also, studies suggest that olive oil, and possibly other monos, can significantly lower blood pressure. Although a little less impressive, polyunsaturates also warrant a place in your diet. They, too, can lower cholesterol levels, but they may also lower HDL in the bargain. No matter which healthy oils you use, be sure to *substitute* them for saturated fats; don't simply add them to your total. And try flavored oils such as chili, sesame, walnut, and hazelnut—just a little goes a long way toward perking up low-fat, low-sodium food.

◇　　　◇　　　◇

Onions: *A family with heart.* Members

of the allium family—onions, leeks, scallions, shallots, and such—are excellent health boosters. They appear to share some of garlic's cholesterol-beating punch. It's even theorized that onions may help offset the artery-clogging effects of a high-fat diet. In addition, certain substances in onions seem to inhibit the formation of blood clots, a principal trigger of most heart attacks. Further, onions, scallions, garlic, and similar bulbous vegetables may guard against the development of stomach cancer.

◇　　　◇　　　◇

Papayas: *Health gift from the*

tropics. Papayas overflow with vitamins A and C. And they're very high in potassium. As a bonus, there's even a portion of bone-building calcium wrapped up in the silky-smooth flesh. A whole papaya contains just 117 calories and would form the basis for a delicious dieter's fruit salad.

◇　　　◇　　　◇

Parsley: *Worth its weight in nutri-*

ents. Parsley is a very-low-cal source of vitamins A and C, potassium, and even calcium, for stronger bones. Throw ½ cup of parsley into your mixed salad, and you get almost half your day's supply of vitamin C and about a third of your vitamin A. With 10 tiny calories in that portion, parsley will certainly help trim your waistline while contributing hunger-satisfying fiber to your diet.

◇　　　◇　　　◇

Parsnips: *Sweet and nutty.* This

old-fashioned relative of the carrot delivers only 63 calories per cooked ½ cup. But its delicious flavor carries with it plenty of potassium plus a little calcium and even vitamin C. And it's got a helping of fiber, which is so important to good health.

◇　　　◇　　　◇

Pasta: *Oodles of benefits.* Once thought

to be fattening, this international favorite has redeemed itself nicely. A 2-ounce serving (about 1 cup cooked) has virtually no fat, just 200 calories, a nice amount of protein, and enough potassium, calcium, iron, and niacin to make it a perfectly healthy food. And pasta retains most of its mineral content after being cooked. Further, dieters and diabetics alike should appreciate pasta's high complex carbohydrates, which can help appease hunger and stabilize blood sugar levels.

◇　　　◇　　　◇

Peaches: *Sweet treat for dieters.*

These juicy fruits should top every dieter's hit parade. With only 37 calories apiece, they're nice sources of fiber, beta-carotene, and potassium.

◇　　　◇　　　◇

Pears: *Boron for the bones.* In addition

to the sterling health-building qualities shared by

many other fruits—few calories, lots of fiber and potassium—pears also contain boron, a trace mineral that may prevent bone-building calcium from being excreted from the body.

◇   ◇   ◇

Peas: Nutrition in a snap. All peas—including the edible-pod varieties—are wonderfully high in dietary fiber, with moderate amounts of potassium and even a nice shot of iron. The edible-pods are higher in vitamin C, especially if eaten raw. But the shelled peas have more vitamin A. Both kinds are extra low in calories. So include both types in your diet to cover all bases.

◇   ◇   ◇

Peppers: Nutrition in many colors. Sweet peppers run the gamut from red and orange to green and purple. But they're all low in calories, fat, and sodium. Red has staggering amounts of vitamins A and C, but the others are still good sources of C. Fiery chili peppers are also healthy food choices. And they may even help prevent heart disease: Hot peppers have been reported to increase the blood's ability to break up potentially dangerous clots. Of further note: Chilies may help burn calories by boosting postmeal metabolism, and they may help relieve congestion, whether due to bronchitis, asthma, allergies, or a cold.

◇   ◇   ◇

Pineapple: Sweet on the stomach—and more. There's more to pineapple than slim calories, high potassium, lots of vitamin C, a helping of fiber, and nice amounts of the trace mineral manganese (essential for protein and calorie metabolism). Scientists say the bromelain enzyme

it contains can aid digestion, attack bacteria, and even help repair damaged skin.

◇   ◇   ◇

Popcorn: Super snack food. Popcorn is a good food for dieters. One cup of crunchy air-popped corn has only 27 calories, a trace of fat, and almost no sodium. In addition, the fiber in popcorn may actually help you *lose* weight. In one study, overweight women lost weight by adding just 6 grams of fiber a day to their diets. That's the amount found in 5 or 6 cups of popcorn.

◇   ◇   ◇

Pork: Lean toward the tenderloin. You may be surprised that pork merits a place in the healthy diet. As with beef and lamb, the cut is the key to healthy eating. Lean tenderloin gets only 26 percent of its calories from fat. That's almost as good as skinless chicken breast (at 20 percent). Center loin, pork leg, lean ham, and Canadian bacon (but not regular bacon) are also good choices. Just trim away all the visible fat. The reason for all this bother is that pork is an excellent source of healing B vitamins, zinc, protein, and iron.

◇   ◇   ◇

Potatoes: Tops in potassium. Potatoes are loaded with potassium, making them a smart choice for those with high blood pressure. They are also good sources of fiber and vitamins C and B_6, with beneficial amounts of iron and magnesium. And they contain virtually no fat. A large baked potato has about 220 calories and can form the centerpiece of any meal when topped with steamed vegetables and yogurt or salsa.

◇   ◇   ◇

RATING THE BIRDS

Here's how various birds compare with one another in terms of calories, grams of fat, and percentage of calories from fat. In all cases, of course, the lower numbers are better. But all the numbers are quite acceptable for a healthy diet. Figures represent 3½ ounces of uncooked boneless meat with both skin and any visible fat removed.

Poultry	Calories	Fat (g)	Calories from Fat (%)
Turkey, fryer-roaster, breast only	111	0.7	5
Capon, breast only	110	1.2	10
Chicken, broiler or fryer, breast only	110	1.2	10
Cornish hen, breast only	110	1.2	10
Turkey, fryer-roaster, light and dark meat	110	1.6	13
Guinea fowl, light and dark meat	110	2.5	20
Chicken, roaster, light and dark meat	111	2.7	21
Turkey, fryer-roaster, dark meat only	111	2.7	21
Quail, breast meat	123	3.0	21
Pheasant, breast meat	133	3.3	22
Chicken, broiler or fryer, light and dark meat	119	3.1	23
Pheasant, light and dark meat	133	3.6	24
Chicken, roaster, dark meat	113	3.6	28
Quail, light and dark meat	134	4.5	30
Capon, dark meat	125	4.3	31
Chicken, broiler or fryer, dark meat	125	4.3	31
Cornish hen, dark meat	125	4.3	31
Duck, wild, breast meat	123	4.3	31

Poultry: *Lean and light.* Turkey and chicken rule the roost when it comes to heart-healthy eating. They contain iron, potassium, B vitamins, and zinc. And they're low in fat and calories (see the chart on the opposite page). For healthiest results, follow a few tips: Don't eat the skin, which is composed largely of fat. Be aware that breast meat is inherently leaner than thigh meat. When preparing thighs and whole birds, remove as much visible fat as possible. As for ground turkey, fat content can vary depending on whether it's made from breast meat or a mixture of light and dark. Read labels or consult your butcher.

◇   ◇   ◇

Prunes: *Nature's laxative.* Prunes are a concentrated storehouse of fiber and nutrients, including vitamin A, potassium, and iron. Their only drawback is a high calorie count, so be sure to cut back elsewhere to make way for these wrinkled wonders.

◇   ◇   ◇

Pumpkin: *A leader in its field.* Pumpkin is overflowing with beta-carotene—½ cup of canned pumpkin has over five times the RDA of vitamin A. That same serving has just 41 calories and a good amount of potassium, plus a helping of iron to help prevent anemia.

◇   ◇   ◇

Quinoa: *Protein pack from the Andes.* This grainlike food was a favorite of the Incans. It is cooked like rice and has a taste reminiscent of squash. With only 159 calories and 2.5 grams of fat per serving, quinoa (pronounced KEEN-wa) makes an excellent grain dish. It also contains an ideal balance of essential amino acids—the National Academy of Sciences dubbed it the best vegetable source of protein. That makes it a good choice for people cutting back on meat and eggs. In addition, it's got calcium, iron, vitamin E, and B vitamins for overall health.

◇   ◇   ◇

Raisins: *Mineral mighty mites.* Like prunes, raisins are a concentrated source of many minerals, including iron and potassium. With virtually no fat, they're perfect for those on a cholesterol-lowering diet. And although they're high in calories, a small handful of raisins has the power to appease a nagging sweet tooth, making dieters less apt to reach for fattening snacks.

◇   ◇   ◇

Rice: *Universal staple of health.* Rice is a terrific complex-carbohydrate food that can satisfy hunger with just a moderate amount of calories—about 115 in ½ cup. This grain is gluten-free and nonallergenic, so it's good for people with those concerns. Best of all, it is incredibly low in fat and sodium and has no cholesterol. With its tan bran intact, brown rice contains quite a bit more fiber than white rice. Rice also contains starch and selenium, both of which may help prevent certain types of cancer.

◇   ◇   ◇

Rutabagas: *Cancer-fighting giants.* Here's another member of the cancer-fighting crucifer family. It's high in potassium, with a good amount of vitamin C and plenty of fiber. But it's low in calories—½ cup of cooked cubes has only 29.

◇   ◇   ◇

Salad greens: *Color is the key.*

Salads are a dieter's mainstay (as long as you use a low-cal dressing). But before you reach for the same old iceberg lettuce, realize that there are plenty of more nutritious greens waiting for a chance to tickle your taste buds. Dark green, leafy vegetables—such as romaine lettuce, chicory, endive, arugula, dandelion and turnip greens—are high in beneficial beta-carotene and vitamin C. Their vibrant color is the clue to their health potential. Greens tend to be so low in calories that you wonder how they can pack so many nutrients. Turnip greens, for instance, have just 7 calories in ½ cup but more than one-fourth of the RDA for vitamin C and an impressive 43 percent of the RDA for vitamin A. Chicory, collards, and dandelion greens have even more of both nutrients. Many greens contain bone-building calcium and cancer-preventing vitamin E. And naturally, these garden greats have plenty of fiber to doubly assure them a place on your plate.

◇   ◇   ◇

Seeds: *Nutritional snack and topping.*

Many seeds, such as anise, dill, fennel, and caraway, rate a place in the healthy diet because they deliver big flavor for virtually no calories. Others, such as sunflower, pumpkin, squash, and sesame, have bigger benefits: Pumpkin seeds contain a nice helping of zinc; sunflower seeds have vitamin E and selenium; sesame seeds sport iron and calcium. Although those larger seeds contain a fair amount of calories and fat, their fat is largely unsaturated—to help prevent heart disease. And seeds in general are high in fiber.

◇   ◇   ◇

Soybeans: *Vegetarian protein plus.*

Soybeans are an excellent source of protein for those cutting back on meat. And they're high in iron, potassium, and calcium. As if that weren't enough, these legumes are loaded with pectin, which has been shown to help lower cholesterol and even to help overeaters stay on their diets.

◇   ◇   ◇

Spinach: *Leaves of plenty.*

One-half cup of cooked spinach has only 21 calories; the same amount raw has just 6. For those few calories, you get plenty of beta-carotene along with fiber, vitamin E, and potassium. One caution: Eating *excessive* amounts of spinach—½ pound a day—can block calcium absorption. But lesser amounts, such as a cup two or three times a week, are just fine.

◇   ◇   ◇

Sprouts: *Protein without calories.*

Most sprouts have more protein than their original seeds, as well as more B vitamins and even vitamin C that the dry seeds don't contain. Sprouts are low in calories: 1 cup of alfalfa sprouts has 10; 1 cup of mung bean sprouts has just 32. And crunchy sprouts give the diet-weary something to chew on.

◇   ◇   ◇

Squash: *Powerhouse of healing.*

Winter squash contains an amazing amount of vitamin A. Just ½ cup of baked butternut or hubbard squash has way more than a full day's supply of this cancer fighter. Squash is also low in calories but high in fiber, with a helping of potassium, vitamin C, calcium, and even iron. Summer squash is less impressive, but it's still extra low in calories, with no fat and a nice amount of fiber.

◇   ◇   ◇

Sweet potatoes: *Bursting with vitamin A.* A single sweet contains more than five times the RDA of vitamin A. Further, sweets contain lots of fiber and vitamin C. And the fiber does double duty to help keep cholesterol levels down and prevent digestive disorders. With a hefty amount of potassium—and hardly any sodium—sweet potatoes are also good for your blood pressure. And with just 114 calories apiece and no fat to speak of, they're a wise choice for dieters.

◇   ◇   ◇

Swiss chard: *Beet-family greens.* Swiss chard is a member of the beet family valued for its large green leaves and celery-like stalks. It's incredibly low in calories (18 in ½ cup of cooked, and just 3 in the same amount raw) but very high in health-boosting vitamin A. It also contains enough fiber and vitamin E to make it a wise addition to your culinary repertoire. And ½ cup of cooked chard has a nice amount of iron, accompanied by a portion of vitamin C to enhance the iron's absorption.

◇   ◇   ◇

Tofu: *Little bundles of soy.* Tofu is a soy product that's very high in good-quality protein, with lots of calcium for strong bones. Unlike the dairy or meat products that it can easily replace, tofu has no cholesterol and contains mostly unsaturated fat. Tofu is also high in iron and potassium but low in sodium. And it even contains fiber—a surprise considering its silken, cheeselike texture.

◇   ◇   ◇

Tomatoes: *The joy of dieting.* Tomatoes are so low in calories that you could eat two a day for the whole summer and never gain an ounce. One whole cup of tomatoes has just 35 calories but lots of potassium, vitamin C, and vitamin A. Don't feel too bad about having to eat canned tomatoes out of season. These beauties contain a bit of calcium and even some iron. If you're concerned about sodium, look for low-salt brands.

◇   ◇   ◇

Tropical fruits: *Tops in taste and nutrition.* When every calorie counts, indulge in a taste of the tropics. These ambrosial fruits have luscious, creamy textures that seem rich and fattening but are really quite low in calories and fat. Further, they tend to be high in vitamins A and C as well as in potassium and fiber. Guavas, for instance, are so packed with vitamin C that a cup of chopped fruit has more than three times as much as an equal amount of orange segments. And that's *five times* the RDA of this infection-fighting nutrient! Passion fruit have just a sprinkling of calories but lots of beneficial fiber, thanks to all their edible seeds. Star fruit have a nice portion of vitamin C plus a helping of vitamin A. And dates, like other dried fruits, are a concentrated source of many vitamins and minerals (but they're also high in calories, so don't go overboard). All of these fruits are good dessert material. And they make wonderful additions to salads of all sorts, including green salads and savory types such as chicken and shrimp.

◇   ◇   ◇

Turnips: *Good for your heart.* As cancer-fighting crucifers, turnips are a good source of fiber and vitamin C. And they're extremely low in calories for a healthy heart and a trimmer profile.

◇   ◇   ◇

Veal: *Better than beef.* Because veal comes from young cattle, it's lower in fat than most cuts of beef. But veal is still high in protein and a very good source of blood-building iron. And it's got plenty of potassium but not too much sodium.

◇   ◇   ◇

Watercress: *Swimming with goodness.* This sprightly green has a pungent flavor with a peppery snap. For practically no calories, you get plenty of beta-carotene plus some calcium, potassium, and vitamin C.

◇   ◇   ◇

Wheat germ: *Nutritional gold.* This cereal food is high in fiber. But it's also a wonderful source of many nutrients, including B vitamins, vitamin E, iron, and potassium. What's more, wheat germ is one of the best sources of zinc. All this with no cholesterol and a reasonable amount of calories and fat (almost all of which is the beneficial unsaturated type). So enjoy wheat germ often. But don't relegate it to the breakfast table. Make it a healthy addition to baked goods, casseroles, salads, and meat loaves.

◇   ◇   ◇

Whole wheat flour: *Foundation of health.* Whole wheat flour has an edge over white: fiber-rich bran. And it retains the nutrient-dense wheat germ (see above) for added health benefits. This flour also contributes B vitamins, vitamin E, iron, potassium, and zinc to a healthy diet. Whole wheat, which tends to be milled more coarsely than white flour, may have an added benefit—studies suggest that finely milled flour triggers a greater insulin surge and may increase the risk of diabetes, atherosclerosis, and obesity.

◇   ◇   ◇

Yogurt: *Cultured to cure.* Dairy products such as low-fat yogurt provide a healthy dose of bone-building calcium. (An 8-ounce serving has more than half the RDA.) But research suggests that this fermented product may offer other benefits, including lower cholesterol and cancer protection. And yogurt is a must for anyone with lactose intolerance. It's got certain enzymes that allow for easy digestion, even if you normally have trouble with dairy products. Yogurt also contains beneficial bacteria that help prevent digestive disorders after antibiotic treatment.

◇   ◇   ◇

CHAPTER TWO ◇

Great Beginnings

T here's a festive aura about appetizers, hors d'oeuvres, and canapés. They evoke images of elegant dinners, intimate soirees, fun-filled parties. And if you feature savory low-fat, high-health starters like the ones that follow, all your gatherings will be cause for celebration.

Red-Pepper Canapés and Carrot Sticks with Dill Pesto, for example, are perfect finger foods. Better yet, they're low in fat and calories. And as a bonus, they're overflowing with beta-carotene, a nutrient that's vital to good health. Savory Stuffed Snow Peas are other hors d'oeuvres that are easy to make and that your guests will relish.

Low-fat, high-protein offerings such as Fragrant Chicken in Bok Choy Leaves let you whet appetites as a first course or satisfy hungry guests at a cocktail party. For nutritious nibbles, provide plenty of crisp raw vegetables with yogurt-based dips such as Sweet and Spicy Curry Dip, Orange-Almond Cheese, and Roasted-Garlic Dip. And scatter bowls of low-fat, high-fiber popcorn wherever guests are likely to congregate. Pesto Popcorn, Curry Popcorn, Chili Popcorn, and Pumpkin-Seed Popcorn are sure winners.

Remember, good times and good health go hand in hand. Get all your special occasions off to the right start.

ARTICHOKE QUICHE

◇ *Per serving*

93 calories
2.5 g. fat
(24% of calories)
3.3 g. dietary fiber
3 mg. cholesterol
112 mg. sodium

3 slices whole wheat bread
1 tablespoon olive oil
1 teaspoon dried thyme
¼ teaspoon paprika
2 cups dry-curd cottage cheese

½ cup egg substitute
2 tablespoons grated Sapsago or Parmesan cheese
12 ounces cooked artichoke hearts

*P*ulverize the bread in a blender or food processor. Transfer to a medium bowl. Add the oil, thyme, and paprika. Press into the bottom and up the sides of a 9-inch pie plate. Bake at 400°F for 7 minutes.

In a food processor, puree the cottage cheese, egg substitute, and Sapsago or Parmesan. Transfer to a large bowl.

Pat the artichokes dry with paper towels. Cut the hearts into bite-size pieces. Stir into the cheese mixture. Pour into the pie shell.

Bake at 350°F for 30 minutes, or until a knife inserted in the center comes out clean. To serve, cut into thin slices.

Serves 8

◇   ◇   ◇

CARROT STICKS WITH DILL PESTO

◇ *Per serving*

72 calories
2 g. fat
(25% of calories)
4.4 g. dietary fiber

2 pounds carrots
3 cloves garlic, halved
1 tablespoon chopped lemon rind

1¾ cups chopped parsley
⅓ cup chopped fresh dill

1 tablespoon olive oil
2 teaspoons lemon juice

0 mg. cholesterol
46 mg. sodium

Cut the carrots into sticks about 3 inches long. Set aside.

In a food processor or blender, process the garlic and lemon rind until minced. Add the parsley and dill. Process until finely minced, stopping to scrape down the sides of the container as needed.

With the motor running, slowly add the oil and blend until a smooth paste is formed. Blend in the lemon juice. Spoon into a serving dish. Serve as a dip for the carrots.

Serves 8

◇　　　　　　◇　　　　　　◇

MUSHROOMS STUFFED WITH CHEESE SOUFFLÉ

◇ *Per serving*

41 calories
0.5 g. fat
(11% of calories)
1.4 g. dietary fiber
<1 mg. cholesterol
38 mg. sodium

1 pound extra-large mushrooms, stems removed	¼ cup dry-curd cottage cheese	¼ teaspoon paprika
1 leek	1 teaspoon Dijon mustard	
	1 egg white	

Blanch the mushrooms in boiling water for about 2 minutes. Remove from the water and drain, stem-side down, while you prepare the filling.

Remove tough green leaves from the leek. Trim the root end and slice the leek in half lengthwise. Rinse well to remove any grit from between the layers. Mince.

In a small bowl, mix the leeks, cottage cheese, and mustard.

In another small bowl, beat the egg white until stiff peaks form. Fold into the cottage cheese mixture.

Spoon the filling into the mushroom caps. Sprinkle with paprika. Bake at 400°F until the filling is set, about 20 minutes.

Serves 6

POPCORN: FLAVORED AND FAVORED

Popcorn's been basted with butter, sprinkled with salt, and slathered with sugar. But beneath all those coatings is a healing food crying to get out. A handful of air-popped popcorn has just 6 tiny little calories. And popcorn is nutritious, too, with a little iron to fight fatigue and some B vitamins to steady nerves.

To make sure your popcorn stays healthy, prepare it yourself. It's a breeze with an electric air popper. If you don't have one, simply use a heavy, deep saucepan. Although popcorn is usually popped over a layer of oil, you can pop it dry. Just place the kernels in the pan, cover with a lid, and pop the corn over high heat. Shake the pan constantly, allowing heat to escape from time to time, until the popping stops.

Keep in mind that ⅓ cup of uncooked kernels makes about 6 to 8 cups of popped corn. Eat your popcorn plain or flavor it with just a sprinkle of oil and a generous shake of herbs or spices. Experiment on your own or try some of these combinations.

◇ ─────────────────────────────

Pesto Popcorn

1 clove garlic, minced	8 cups popped corn
1 teaspoon olive oil	1 tablespoon grated Parmesan cheese
½ teaspoon dried basil	
½ teaspoon dried parsley	

In a 4-quart saucepan, cook the garlic in the oil for 1 minute (don't brown). Stir in the basil and parsley. Add the popcorn and mix well. Sprinkle with the cheese and mix well.

Makes 8 cups

◇*Per cup:* 34 calories, 0.8 g. fat (21% of calories), 0.4 g. dietary fiber, <1 mg. cholesterol, 15 mg. sodium

◇ ─────────────────────────────

Curry Popcorn

2 teaspoons curry powder	8 cups popped corn
2 teaspoons canola oil	

In a 4-quart saucepan, heat the curry powder in the oil until fragrant. Add the popcorn and mix well.

Makes 8 cups

◇ *Per cup:* *31 calories, 0.6 g. fat (17% of calories), 0.5 g. dietary fiber, 0 mg. cholesterol, 0 mg. sodium*

◇ ───────────────────────────────

Pumpkin-Seed Popcorn

2 tablespoons pumpkin seeds	⅛ teaspoon chili powder
1 teaspoon canola oil	⅛ teaspoon ground cumin
¼ teaspoon dried oregano	8 cups popped corn

In a 4-quart saucepan over low heat, lightly toast the pumpkin seeds in the oil, stirring frequently. Stir in the oregano, chili powder, and cumin. Add the popcorn and mix well.

Makes 8 cups

◇ *Per cup:* *37 calories, 1 g. fat (24% of calories), 0.6 g. dietary fiber, 0 mg. cholesterol, 1 mg. sodium*

◇ ───────────────────────────────

Chili Popcorn

1 tablespoon tomato paste	1 teaspoon chili powder
1 teaspoon canola oil	8 cups popped corn
2 tablespoons water	

In a 1-quart saucepan, combine the tomato paste and oil. Stir over medium heat for 1 minute. Add the water and chili powder. Cook for 2 minutes. Drizzle over the popcorn and mix well.

Makes 8 cups

◇ *Per cup:* *33 calories, 0.6 g. fat (16% of calories), 0.6 g. dietary fiber, 0 mg. cholesterol, 5 mg. sodium*

RED PEPPER CANAPÉS

◇ *Per serving*

190 calories
5.3 g. fat
(25% of calories)
3.1 g. dietary fiber
0 mg. cholesterol
484 mg. sodium

5 sweet red peppers, cut into ½-inch strips
1 eggplant, cubed
¼ cup defatted stock
2 tablespoons olive oil
1½ cups tomato sauce
1 onion, sliced

1 carrot, finely chopped
1 stalk celery, finely chopped
1 cup sliced mushrooms
3 cloves garlic, minced
1 bay leaf
½ teaspoon dried oregano

½ teaspoon dried thyme
1 tablespoon red-wine vinegar
1 tablespoon lemon juice
1 loaf whole wheat French bread, thinly sliced

*I*n a 4-quart pot, sauté the peppers and eggplant in the stock and oil until tender, about 10 to 15 minutes. Set aside.

In a 2-quart saucepan, combine the tomato sauce, onions, carrots, celery, mushrooms, garlic, bay leaf, oregano, and thyme. Simmer over medium heat until the vegetables are tender, about 20 minutes.

Add the vinegar, lemon juice, and peppers and eggplant. Stir to combine. Chill. Discard the bay leaf.

Serve the vegetables on slices of French bread.

Serves 8

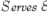

BRAISED LEEKS
WITH MUSTARD SAUCE

◇ *Per serving*

73 calories
0.5 g. fat

1 pound thin leeks
1 cup defatted chicken stock

¼ teaspoon yellow mustard seeds

1 bay leaf
1½ teaspoons Dijon mustard

(6% of calories)
2.3 g. dietary fiber
0 mg. cholesterol
71 mg. sodium

Slice off the roots and tough green parts of the leeks. Then rinse the leeks carefully to remove all sand and grit. If the leeks are less than 1 inch in diameter, leave them whole. Otherwise, cut in half lengthwise, taking care not to disrupt the layers.

Combine the stock, mustard seeds, and bay leaf in a large frying pan. Add the leeks, cut-side down. Bring to a simmer over medium heat. Then cover the pan and simmer for 8 minutes.

Remove the lid and set the pan in the refrigerator for about 30 minutes to chill.

When ready to serve, arrange the leeks on a serving platter. Strain and reserve the stock.

To make the mustard sauce, combine 3 tablespoons of the reserved stock with the Dijon mustard. Drizzle over the leeks.

Serves 4

MICRO METHOD: Is Your Dishware Safe?

A microwave can be a great timesaver when cooking for a crowd. Hot dishes can be prepared in advance and arranged on their serving plates. Then it takes only a few minutes to zap them in the microwave and get them to the buffet table, still piping hot.

Glass, china, paper, pottery, and certain plastics commonly used for entertaining are also appropriate materials for the microwave. But check beforehand to make sure they are microwave safe. Look for labels that say "microwave oven safe" or "suitable for microwave." Make sure that dishes, teapots, and other items have no metal trim or screws in the handles or lids.

If you're unsure whether a piece of cookware is suitable for microwaving, perform this test.

- Fill a glass measuring cup with 1 cup of water.
- Place it in the microwave on or next to the dish you wish to test.
- Run the microwave for 1 minute on full power.
- If the dish becomes hot, don't use it for microwaving. Only the water in the cup should heat up.

Spinach-Stuffed Mushrooms

◇ *Per serving*

83 calories
2.2 g. fat
(24% of calories)
2.9 g. dietary fiber
3 mg. cholesterol
184 mg. sodium

10 ounces spinach
1½ pounds extra-large mushrooms
½ cup minced onions
1 teaspoon olive oil

1 cup dry-curd cottage cheese
2 tablespoons grated Parmesan cheese
1 teaspoon dillweed

1 tablespoon low-sodium soy sauce
¼ teaspoon ground pepper

Wash the spinach in plenty of cold water to remove any grit. Remove thick stems. Transfer the spinach to a large pot with just the water left clinging to the leaves. Cover and cook until wilted, about 5 minutes. Drain and let cool. Squeeze out excess moisture and chop finely.

Carefully separate the stems from the mushroom caps. Place the caps, stem-side up, in an oiled baking dish.

In a large nonstick frying pan, sauté the onions in the oil until soft.

Finely chop the mushroom stems and add to the pan with the onions. Sauté for 3 minutes. Remove from the heat and stir in the spinach, cottage cheese, Parmesan, dill, soy sauce, and pepper.

Divide the mixture among the mushroom caps, mounding it. Bake at 400°F for 20 minutes, or until the tops are lightly browned.

Serves 6

Fragrant Chicken in Bok Choy Leaves

◇ *Per bundle*

35 calories
0.9 g. fat
(23% of calories)
1.1 g. dietary fiber
9 mg. cholesterol
41 mg. sodium

1 pound boneless, skinless chicken breasts
¼ cup minced scallions
1 tablespoon tahini (sesame-seed paste)
1 tablespoon low-sodium soy sauce
1 tablespoon peeled minced gingerroot
2 cloves garlic, minced
1 teaspoon lemon juice
1 teaspoon honey
24 bok choy leaves

Cut the chicken into 1-inch pieces. Transfer to a food processor and mince with on/off turns. Add the scallions, tahini, soy sauce, ginger, garlic, lemon juice, and honey. Process until just combined.

Place a rounded tablespoon of chicken mixture on the long edge of each bok choy leaf. Roll up, tucking in the corners as you go, to form cylindrical bundles.

Steam until the filling is cooked, about 10 minutes. (If necessary, steam in batches.)

Makes 24

BETTER THAN CREAM CHEESE

Make your own lusciously smooth, creamy, low-fat alternative to cream cheese. It's called yogurt cheese, and it's got a lot going for it: just a fraction of cream cheese's calories and—if you use nonfat yogurt—none of its fat. Best of all, it's a snap to make.

Just line a large strainer with cheesecloth, white paper towels, or a coffee filter. (Or use a special yogurt-cheese funnel.) Spoon in 4 cups of plain nonfat yogurt and let the whey drain out overnight. You'll end up with 1½ to 2 cups of nonfat yogurt cheese. Store your cheese covered in the refrigerator.

One note: Some brands of yogurt have gelatin or stabilizers in them that prevent the whey from draining off. Reading the label isn't always enough to tell you whether a particular yogurt is drainable. So try this test at home: Take a big spoonful of yogurt out of the container, leaving a depression. If the hole starts to fill with liquid within 10 minutes, you should have success making yogurt cheese.

Here are some ways to use your yogurt cheese for canapés on your hors d'oeuvre tray.

- Fold in chives and use to top baked potato slices or potato skins.
- Add fresh or dried herbs and use as a savory spread for toast or crackers.
- Mix with minced smoked turkey and use in place of cream cheese on bagel crisps.
- Stir in orange juice concentrate and minced fruit (such as strawberries) and use as a topping on cheese and crackers.
- Mix with Mexican salsa and use as a dip for crisp raw vegetables.

◇ ——————————————————

Sweet and Spicy Curry Dip

¼ cup fruit chutney	1 cup nonfat yogurt cheese
1 tablespoon curry powder	⅛ teaspoon hot-pepper sauce

In a 1-quart saucepan, heat the chutney and curry powder for 1 minute, stirring frequently. Cool slightly.

In a small bowl, combine the yogurt cheese, curry mixture, and hot-pepper sauce.

Makes about 1 cup

◇*Per tablespoon: 23 calories, 0.1 g. fat (4% of calories), 0.1 g. dietary fiber, 0 mg. cholesterol, 2 mg. sodium*

Roasted-Garlic Dip

8 cloves garlic,
  unpeeled
⅓ cup water
1 bay leaf
1 cup nonfat
  yogurt cheese

⅛ teaspoon
  ground red
  pepper

Place the garlic in a small ovenproof dish. Add the water and bay leaf. Bake at 350°F for 25 to 35 minutes, or until the garlic is tender. Discard the bay leaf.

Squeeze each clove of garlic out of its skin. Place in a small dish and mash well. Stir in the yogurt cheese and pepper.

Makes about 1 cup

◇*Per tablespoon:* 14 calories, 0.1 g. fat (<1% of calories), 0 g. dietary fiber, 0 mg. cholesterol, 1 mg. sodium

---

◇

Orange-Almond Cheese

1 cup nonfat
  yogurt cheese
3 tablespoons
  raisins, minced
1 tablespoon
  chopped
  almonds
1½ teaspoons
  honey

1½ teaspoons
  orange juice
  concentrate
⅛ teaspoon
  ground
  cinnamon

In a medium bowl, combine the yogurt cheese, raisins, almonds, honey, juice, and cinnamon.

Makes about 1 cup

◇*Per tablespoon:* 23 calories, 0.3 g. fat (12% of calories), 0.1 g. dietary fiber, 0 mg. cholesterol, 1 mg. sodium

ONION TOAST

◇ *Per serving*

193 calories
4.4 g. fat
(21% of calories)
5.7 g. dietary fiber
<1 mg. cholesterol
43 mg. sodium

1 tablespoon olive oil
1 teaspoon honey
1 teaspoon low-sodium soy sauce

¼ teaspoon ground red pepper
2½ pounds onions, thinly sliced
¼ cup apple-cider vinegar

½ teaspoon dried thyme
1 loaf whole wheat French bread, thinly sliced

*I*n a large nonstick frying pan over medium heat, combine the oil, honey, soy sauce, and pepper.

Add the onions and stir to combine. Cover the pan and simmer over medium-low heat for 30 minutes, stirring occasionally.

Stir in the vinegar and thyme. Cover and simmer for about 20 minutes, stirring occasionally, until the onions are very soft and thick, having absorbed all the liquid.

While the onions are cooking, place the bread slices in a single layer on cookie sheets. Bake at 350°F for about 10 minutes per side to toast lightly.

Spread the slices with the warm onion mixture.

Serves 8

WATERCRESS CANAPÉS

◇ *Per serving*

77 calories
1.2 g. fat
(14% of calories)
3.3 g. dietary fiber

1 cup nonfat yogurt
2 scallions, minced
1 teaspoon dillweed

12 slices whole-grain bread
2 cups thinly sliced cucumbers

4 cups watercress sprigs
12 radishes, thinly sliced

great beginnings

<1 mg. cholesterol
180 mg. sodium

Spoon the yogurt into a strainer lined with cheesecloth. Place over a bowl and allow to drain until thick, about 4 hours. Transfer to a small bowl and stir in the scallions and dill.

If desired, trim the crusts from the bread. Spread the bread with the yogurt mixture. Divide the cucumbers, watercress, and radishes among the slices and arrange them in attractive layers on the yogurt mixture.

Cut each slice into four squares or triangles.

Serves 12

◇   ◇   ◇

VEGETABLES WITH CREAMY GARLIC SAUCE

◇ *Per serving*

293 calories
4.8 g. fat
(15% of calories)
7.3 g. dietary fiber
1 mg. cholesterol
135 mg. sodium

1 cup nonfat yogurt
6 cloves garlic, minced
1 tablespoon olive oil
1 large artichoke, cooked and cooled

8 small potatoes, halved and steamed
1 cup carrot sticks, blanched
8 small beets, cooked and cooled

1 cup cooked chick-peas

In a small bowl, fold together the yogurt, garlic, and olive oil. Transfer to a small serving bowl.

Arrange the artichoke, potatoes, carrots, beets, and chick-peas on a large platter.

Serve the vegetables with the sauce. (Eat the artichoke by tearing off leaves and dipping them into the sauce.)

Serves 4

Savory Stuffed Snow Peas

◇ *Per serving*

37 calories
0.1 g. fat
(2% of calories)
0.4 g. dietary fiber
1 mg. cholesterol
40 mg. sodium

4 cloves garlic
2 cups nonfat
  yogurt
1 teaspoon
  dillweed

1 teaspoon
  dried savory
36 snow peas

*B*oil the garlic for 2 minutes, then mash to a paste.

In a medium bowl, mix the garlic, yogurt, dill, and savory. Pour into a strainer lined with cheesecloth. Cover with a piece of plastic set over a bowl, and allow the yogurt to drain overnight. (Refrigerate in warm weather.)

Boil the snow peas for 2 minutes. Drain and cool. Open one long side of each pod.

Using a small spoon or a pastry bag fitted with a star tip, fill each pod with the yogurt mixture.

Serves 9

Horseradish Dip

◇ *Per tablespoon*

7 calories
<0.1 g. fat
(3% of calories)
0 g. dietary fiber
0 mg. cholesterol
24 mg. sodium

1 ½ cups nonfat
  yogurt
½ cup minced
  scallions

3 tablespoons
  prepared
  horseradish

2 tablespoons
  snipped
  chives

*I*n a small bowl, combine the yogurt, scallions, horseradish, and chives.

Makes 2 cups

CHAPTER THREE ◇

Soups and Chowders

Soup made a stir in the research lab a few years back when scientists discovered that eating it can help you lose weight. It's been a hot issue ever since.

In one study, for example, researchers asked dieters to eat soup with one or more meals a day. After one year, the soup group wound up considerably slimmer than another group of dieters who ate the same number of calories, but without the daily soup requirement. What does soup have that makes it such choice diet fare? For starters, theorize researchers, soup tends to be eaten hot. That means you consume it slowly, giving your appetite time to be satisfied before you can overeat. Also, soup is made up largely of water, and its bulk consists mainly of low-calorie vegetables plus fiber-rich grains and legumes—all of which can fill you up without filling you out.

Every recipe in this chapter was created with that mission in mind. And many—such as Striper Chowder and Eight-Vegetable Millet Soup—are so hearty that they can stand alone as a meal. You'll even find you can enjoy creamy varieties without using high-fat butter, eggs, cream, or milk. "Getting Great Body" on page 43 tells you how.

Even fruit has found a place in the soup pot. Cool Peach Soup, Iced Cantaloupe Soup, and Chilled Blueberry Soup are excellent cool trade-offs for hot summer days.

EGGPLANT SOUP WITH TINY PASTA

1 large onion, minced
½ cup minced celery
3 cloves garlic, minced
2 teaspoons olive oil
2 cups cubed eggplant

2 cups chopped tomatoes
1¾ cups defatted chicken stock
⅛ teaspoon dried thyme
⅛ teaspoon crushed rosemary

½ cup orzo or other tiny pasta, cooked

*I*n a 3-quart saucepan over medium heat, sauté the onions, celery, and garlic in the oil for 3 minutes.

Add the eggplant and tomatoes. Cover and simmer for 10 minutes.

Add the stock, thyme, and rosemary. Simmer for 20 minutes. Add the pasta and heat through.

Serves 4

STRIPER CHOWDER

12 ounces striped-bass fillets
⅓ cup thinly sliced scallions
1 tablespoon olive oil
1 teaspoon minced garlic

3 cups defatted stock
1 cup chopped tomatoes
1 cup cubed potatoes
2 teaspoons prepared horseradish

1 teaspoon lemon juice
½ teaspoon dried thyme
⅛ teaspoon red pepper
2 bay leaves
1 cup cooked rice
½ cup minced fresh parsley

Cut the bass into ½-inch chunks and set aside.

In a 3-quart saucepan over medium heat, sauté the scallions in the oil for 5 minutes. Add the garlic and sauté for 1 minute.

Add the stock, tomatoes, potatoes, horseradish, lemon juice, thyme, red pepper, and bay leaves.

Bring to a boil, then lower the heat and simmer for 10 minutes.

Add the fish, rice, and parsley. Simmer for 5 minutes. Discard the bay leaves.

Serves 4

◇　　　　　　　　　◇　　　　　　　　　◇

DILLED CABBAGE SOUP

½ medium cabbage, chopped
2 large onions, chopped
1 teaspoon dill seeds
½ teaspoon caraway seeds

1 tablespoon olive oil
4 cloves garlic, minced
1 tablespoon vinegar
3 cups defatted stock
1½ cups tomato juice

1 large potato, diced
2 teaspoons low-sodium soy sauce
¼ cup minced fresh parsley

In a 3-quart saucepan, sauté the cabbage, onions, dill, and caraway in the oil, stirring occasionally, until the cabbage is translucent and wilted, about 10 minutes.

Add the garlic and vinegar. Cook for 1 minute. Add the stock, tomato juice, potatoes, and soy sauce.

Cover and simmer until the potatoes are tender, about 15 to 20 minutes. Add the parsley.

Serves 4

PUMPKIN SOUP

1 large onion,
  minced
2 cups defatted
  chicken stock
1½ cups pureed
  cooked
  pumpkin
½ teaspoon
  dried
  oregano

¼ teaspoon
  hot-pepper
  sauce
¼ cup toasted
  pumpkin
  seeds

*I*n a 2-quart saucepan, cook the onions in 2 tablespoons of the stock until limp.

Add the remaining stock, pumpkin, oregano, and hot-pepper sauce. Simmer for 15 minutes.

Serve sprinkled with pumpkin seeds.

Serves 4

◇

ESCAROLE SOUP

4 cups defatted
  chicken stock
1½ cups diced
  onions
1 cup diced
  celery

1 cup thinly
  sliced carrots
1 cup thinly
  sliced
  parsnips
½ teaspoon
  curry powder

¼ teaspoon
  ground
  fennel
1½ cups
  chopped
  escarole

*I*n a 3-quart saucepan, combine the stock, onions, celery, carrots, parsnips, curry powder, and fennel. Bring to a boil, then reduce the heat and simmer until the vegetables are tender, about 30 minutes.

Add the escarole and cook for 10 minutes.

Serves 4

soups and chowders

MICRO METHOD: Fresh-Tasting Soups

Microwaving enhances the flavor of vegetables, yielding soups that taste fresher than conventionally cooked potages. Use these guidelines to convert your favorite recipes to the microwave.

■ Reduce the amount of liquid in your conventional recipe by one-fourth, since very little liquid evaporates during the short time it takes for microwaving soup. Exceptions are soups made with dried peas or beans. These need the full amount of liquid to rehydrate the legumes. (And some of the water *will* evaporate during the longer microwaving time needed for these types of soup.)

■ Cut meat and vegetables into small, uniform pieces so they'll cook evenly and quickly.

■ Microwave clear soups or brothy chicken-and-vegetable soups on high power.

■ Use medium (50 percent) power and longer cooking times for soups based on less tender cuts of meats, such as beef cubes. Start by cooking the beef in liquid to cover until tender. Then add vegetables and seasonings.

■ For chicken stews, use broiler-fryers. They're younger and more tender than stewing hens. (You can microwave stewing hens, but they'll take nearly as long as with conventional cooking methods. Use medium power.)

■ When making fish or shellfish soups, cook the rest of the ingredients first. Seafood begins to cook as soon as it's added to hot liquid. To avoid overcooking these delicate items, use 50 percent power and cook just until opaque. Allow a few minutes' standing time after microwaving to complete the cooking process.

■ Soups or chowders made with milk can be microwaved on high. Choose a container that will hold double the volume of soup you are microwaving to avoid boil-overs.

■ When precooking vegetables for pureed soups, use high power and little or no liquid.

■ Making very thick pureed soups is easy in the microwave. Conventional thick soups made on the stove must be cooked over low heat and stirred often to prevent sticking. Since sticking is not a problem with the microwave, such soups can be cooked on high and stirred only two or three times throughout cooking.

ICED CANTALOUPE SOUP

◇ *Per serving*

134 calories
2.2 g. fat
(15% of calories)
1.1 g. dietary fiber
7 mg. cholesterol
81 mg. sodium

1 large cantaloupe	¾ teaspoon ground cinnamon	½ cup nonfat yogurt
1½ cups low-fat milk	¾ teaspoon ground coriander	
2 tablespoons maple syrup		

*R*emove the seeds and rind from the cantaloupe. Cut the flesh into cubes.

In a blender, combine the cantaloupe, milk, maple syrup, cinnamon, and coriander. Blend well.

Transfer to a large bowl. Cover and chill for 1 hour.

While the soup is chilling, spoon the yogurt into a cheesecloth-lined sieve. Let drain over a bowl to thicken.

Whisk the yogurt into the soup.

Serves 4

◇ ◇

CREAM OF CARROT SOUP

◇ *Per serving*

117 calories
1.8 g. fat
(14% of calories)
2.8 g. dietary fiber
<1 mg. cholesterol
51 mg. sodium

1 large onion, sliced	2 cups defatted stock	1 large potato, cubed
1 teaspoon canola oil	4 ounces carrots, sliced	½ teaspoon dried thyme
		¾ cup skim milk

*I*n a 2-quart saucepan, sauté the onions in the oil until softened, about 5 minutes.

Add the stock, carrots, potatoes, and thyme. Simmer until tender, about 25 minutes.

Puree in a food mill or blender. Stir in the milk.

Serves 4

Garlic and Potato Soup

◇ *Per serving*

247 calories
2.5 g. fat
(9% of calories)
4.1 g. dietary fiber
9 mg. cholesterol
193 mg. sodium

2 medium leeks
3 cups defatted stock
1 pound potatoes, cubed

4 cloves garlic, minced
1 cup evaporated skim milk

¼ cup snipped chives
2 tablespoons crumbled feta cheese

*R*emove and discard the tough green leaves and root end of the leeks. Cut the leeks in half lengthwise. Wash well to remove any dirt from between the layers, then slice thinly.

In a 3-quart saucepan, combine the leeks, stock, potatoes, and garlic. Bring to a boil. Reduce the heat to medium-low, cover loosely, and simmer until the potatoes are tender, about 15 minutes.

Stir in the milk and chives. Simmer just until heated through.

Place the cheese in a strainer. Rinse with cold water to remove excess salt. Pat dry. Sprinkle over the soup.

Serves 4

Cold Zucchini Soup

◇ *Per serving*

68 calories
0.7 g. fat
(9% of calories)
4.3 g. dietary fiber
0 mg. cholesterol
36 mg. sodium

8 tomatoes, quartered
2 medium zucchini, chopped
3 stalks celery, chopped
1 green pepper, quartered

1 large onion, quartered
2 tablespoons lemon juice
½ teaspoon dried basil

½ teaspoon ground cumin
½ teaspoon grated lemon rind

*I*n a food processor, combine the tomatoes, zucchini, celery, peppers, onions, lemon juice, basil, cumin, and lemon rind. Process with on/off turns until smooth. Served chilled.

Serves 6

CAJUN SOUP

◇ *Per serving*

230 calories
4.6 g. fat
(18% of calories)
6.1 g. dietary fiber
0 mg. cholesterol
70 mg. sodium

1 large onion, chopped
1 tablespoon olive oil
1 green pepper, diced
½ cup chopped celery
3 cloves garlic, minced
4 cups defatted chicken stock

1 large tomato, chopped
2 bay leaves
½ teaspoon dried rosemary
½ teaspoon dried oregano
½ teaspoon dried basil
4 cups corn

1 cup shredded Swiss chard
½ cup cooked black-eyed peas
¾ teaspoon paprika
¼ teaspoon red pepper
¼ teaspoon black pepper

*I*n a 4-quart pot over medium heat, sauté the onions in the oil until light brown, 7 to 8 minutes. Add the green peppers, celery, and garlic. Cook for 5 minutes.

Add the stock, tomatoes, bay leaves, rosemary, oregano, and basil. Bring to a boil. Cover and simmer 15 minutes.

Add the corn, Swiss chard, black-eyed peas, paprika, and red and black pepper. Simmer for 5 minutes. Discard the bay leaves.

Serves 4

COOL PEACH SOUP

◇ *Per serving*

188 calories
0.6 g. fat
(3% of calories)
4.1 g. dietary fiber
0 mg. cholesterol
16 mg. sodium

1 cup white grape juice
1 cup water
⅓ cup apple juice concentrate
1 teaspoon vanilla extract

¼ teaspoon ground cinnamon
2 teaspoons lemon juice
4 large peaches
1 pint raspberries

*I*n a 1-quart saucepan, bring the grape juice, water, apple juice concentrate, vanilla, and cinnamon to a boil. Simmer for 2 minutes.

Remove the pan from the heat and stir in the lemon juice.

Peel the peaches by immersing them in boiling water for about 1 minute, then running them under cold water. The skins will easily slip off.

Chop two of the peaches and place in a blender or food processor. Add the liquid and process until smooth. Transfer to a large bowl.

Cut the remaining peaches into ½-inch wedges. Add to the bowl, making sure the slices are covered with puree so they won't discolor.

Refrigerate the soup for at least 1 hour, or until well chilled.

Serve in shallow bowls topped with raspberries.

Serves 4

◇   ◇   ◇

GETTING GREAT BODY

Give your soups the rich, thick, satisfying texture you crave without resorting to butter, egg yolks, and cream. Simply puree part of the batch and add it back to the pot. Or stir in one or more of the following ingredients.

- Mashed potatoes
- Pureed vegetables, such as carrots, corn, or onions
- Evaporated skim milk
- Buttermilk
- Rice (whole or pureed)
- Beans (mash all or part of them)
- Pasta
- Bread cubes

CHILLED BLUEBERRY SOUP

◇ *Per serving*

115 calories
0.4 g. fat
(3% of calories)
1.9 g. dietary fiber
1 mg. cholesterol
41 mg. sodium

2 cups
  blueberries
¾ cup apple
  juice
¼ cup orange
  juice

¼ teaspoon
  lemon extract
⅛ teaspoon
  grated nutmeg
1 cup nonfat
  vanilla yogurt

*I*n a 2-quart saucepan, combine the blueberries, apple juice, orange juice, lemon extract, and nutmeg. Bring to a boil over medium heat, stirring occasionally.

Reduce the heat and simmer for 1 minute.

Let cool for 5 minutes. Transfer to a blender and puree until smooth. Transfer to a large bowl. Chill for 1 hour.

While the soup is chilling, spoon the yogurt into cheesecloth-lined sieve. Let drain over a bowl to thicken.

To serve, ladle the soup into individual bowls. Top with dollops of yogurt.

Serves 4

◇   ◇   ◇

SWEETHEART SOUP

◇ *Per serving*

85 calories
2.2 g. fat
(23% of calories)
2.6 g. dietary fiber
<1 mg. cholesterol
49 mg. sodium

8 sweet red
  peppers,
  chopped
½ cup minced
  celery
2 cloves garlic,
  minced
2 shallots,
  minced
1 tablespoon
  peeled minced
  gingerroot

1 teaspoon
  olive oil
4 cups defatted
  chicken stock
1 tablespoon
  lime juice
¼ teaspoon
  ground
  coriander

⅛ teaspoon
  ground ginger
1 tablespoon
  nonfat yogurt
1 tablespoon
  evaporated
  skim milk

In a 3-quart saucepan, sauté the peppers, celery, garlic, shallots, and minced ginger in the oil for 5 minutes.

Add the stock, lime juice, coriander, and ground ginger. Simmer for 25 to 30 minutes, or until the peppers are tender. Let cool about 5 minutes.

In a blender, puree the soup in batches until smooth.

Pour into individual bowls.

To make the hearts, mix the yogurt and milk in a cup. Place a dot (about ¼ teaspoon) of the mixture on the surface of one bowl of soup. Place a toothpick in the soup about ¼ inch away from the dot and draw it through the dot, lifting it when the tail of the heart is about ½ inch long. Wipe off the toothpick. Repeat to make several hearts in each bowl.

Serves 4

◇　　　　　　　　　　　◇　　　　　　　　　　　◇

Fragrant Borscht

4 cups defatted beef stock	¼ cup vinegar	1½ cups nonfat yogurt
4 large beets, peeled and shredded	2 tablespoons honey	
½ medium cabbage, shredded	2 teaspoons low-sodium soy sauce	
	½ cup tomato puree	

In a 3-quart saucepan, combine the stock and beets. Cover and cook over medium heat until tender, about 20 to 25 minutes.

Add the cabbage, vinegar, honey, and soy sauce. Cover and cook until the cabbage begins to soften, about 7 to 10 minutes.

Add the tomato puree and cook 10 to 15 minutes.

To serve, ladle into soup bowls and top with a large spoonful of yogurt.

Serves 4

CREAMY BROCCOLI SOUP

1 large onion, diced
1 teaspoon olive oil
2 cups defatted stock
1 pound broccoli florets, chopped
1 cup cooked white beans
1 bay leaf
¼ teaspoon ground allspice

*I*n a 3-quart saucepan, sauté the onions in the oil until brown, about 15 minutes. Add the stock, broccoli, beans, bay leaf, and allspice. Bring to a boil.

Reduce the heat to a simmer, partially cover, and simmer until the broccoli is tender, about 20 minutes.

Let cool for 5 minutes. Discard the bay leaf.

In a food processor or blender, puree the soup.

Serves 4

◇ ◇

BROCCOLI-BUTTERMILK SOUP

1 pound broccoli florets
1 cup sliced onions
4 cloves garlic
2 cups buttermilk

*C*ombine the broccoli, onions, and garlic in a steamer basket. Steam over boiling water until the broccoli is tender, about 12 minutes.

Transfer the vegetables to a food processor or blender and blend until pureed. Stir in the buttermilk.

Serves 4

SALMON BISQUE

◇ *Per serving*

163 calories
4.6 g. fat
(25% of calories)
2 g. dietary fiber
15 mg. cholesterol
527 mg. sodium

1 large onion, diced
2 teaspoons olive oil
2 tablespoons flour
2½ cups defatted stock

1½ cups tomato puree
1 pound salmon fillet, cut into ½-inch chunks

2 tablespoons minced fresh parsley
2 cups evaporated skim milk

*I*n a 3-quart saucepan, sauté the onions in the oil until translucent, about 5 minutes. Add the flour and cook until light brown, about 3 minutes.

Add the stock, tomato puree, salmon, and parsley. Simmer for 10 minutes.

Add the milk and heat through.

Serves 6

◇

SAFETY FIRST

Bacteria love a good batch of stock as much as you do. They make themselves at home, prosper, and multiply. That's fine for them but potentially dangerous for you. So you need to handle your finished stock in a way that discourages bacterial growth. Here's how.

■ Cool your finished stock quickly—and completely—before storing. Otherwise, warm stock at the center of the container will be just the right temperature for bacteria to thrive, even in the refrigerator.

■ The easiest way to cool stock is to set the pot in a larger container of ice water. If the pot is very big, use your sink. (But be careful not to tip the stock pot, or the ice water will dilute your perfectly seasoned stock.)

■ Refrigerate only as much stock as you can use within a few days. Freeze the rest in pint or quart containers. (Be sure to label and date the containers and to use the stock within six months.)

■ Before using your stock—whether frozen or refrigerated—bring it to a rolling boil as an extra precaution against bacteria.

Irish Vichyssoise

◇ *Per serving*

341 calories
2.4 g. fat
(6% of calories)
9 g. dietary fiber
5 mg. cholesterol
213 mg. sodium

3 large potatoes, diced
1 large bunch broccoli, chopped
1 large onion, sliced
1 teaspoon olive oil
½ teaspoon dried thyme

¼ teaspoon ground rosemary
¼ teaspoon ground cumin
2 cups evaporated skim milk
1 cup defatted stock

Steam the potatoes and broccoli for 10 minutes, or until tender.

In a 3-quart saucepan, sauté the onions in the oil for 5 minutes. Add the thyme, rosemary, and cumin. Cook for 1 minute.

In a blender, working in batches, puree the potatoes, broccoli, and onions with the milk and stock. Return the soup to the saucepan and heat through.

Serves 4

◇ ◇ ◇

Creamy Corn Chowder

◇ *Per serving*

386 calories
7.6 g. fat
(18% of calories)
10 g. dietary fiber
2 mg. cholesterol
135 mg. sodium

1 sweet red pepper, diced
½ cup minced scallions
1 tablespoon olive oil
1 tablespoon whole wheat flour

2 cups corn
1¾ cups skim milk
1 teaspoon low-sodium soy sauce
⅛ teaspoon grated nutmeg

soups and chowders

In a 2-quart saucepan over medium heat, sauté the peppers and scallions in the oil until crisp-tender, about 3 minutes.

Add the flour and cook 1 to 2 minutes more, stirring constantly. Remove from the heat.

In a blender, puree 1 cup of corn with 1 cup of milk. Add to the saucepan. Add the remaining corn and milk, soy sauce, and nutmeg.

Cook over medium heat, stirring frequently, until hot but not boiling. Reduce the heat and simmer for 5 minutes.

Serves 4

◇   ◇   ◇

EIGHT-VEGETABLE MILLET SOUP

◇ *Per serving*

170 calories
3.5 g. fat
(19% of calories)
5.4 g. dietary fiber
1 mg. cholesterol
62 mg. sodium

1 large onion, diced
1 tablespoon olive oil
3 cups defatted chicken stock
2 carrots, diced
1 large potato, diced
1 stalk celery, diced

1 zucchini, chopped
1 cup sliced green beans
1 tomato, diced
1 bay leaf
½ teaspoon dried thyme

½ teaspoon dried basil
1 cup shredded spinach
1 cup cooked millet
1 cup skim milk

In a 3-quart saucepan, sauté the onions in the oil until translucent.

Add the stock, carrots, potatoes, celery, zucchini, beans, tomatoes, bay leaf, thyme, and basil. Simmer for 30 minutes.

Stir in the spinach, millet, and milk. Simmer for 5 minutes. Discard the bay leaf.

Serves 6

CHAPTER FOUR ◇

The Super Salad Bowl

*I*f your idea of a green salad is a wedge of iceberg lettuce, it's time to break out of the pale green rut. Just follow the green rule of thumb: The more colorful a salad ingredient, the more nutritious it is. Deep green romaine lettuce, for example, has *eight times* more vitamin A than iceberg!

Other good choices include silky butterhead lettuce, deep-lobed oakleaf lettuce, fringed endive, emerald green spinach, arugula, watercress, hearty Swiss chard, and kale. And don't forget red radicchio! This ruby red jewel can add color and nutrients to salads when the only fresh tomatoes on the market are as hard as golf balls.

Supermarkets, farmers' markets, and your own garden are wonderful sources of healthy salad fixings. But don't stop with lettuce. Cruciferous vegetables such as broccoli, cauliflower, and bok choy (Chinese cabbage) add crunch, texture, and fiber to salads—and they may help protect against certain kinds of cancer. Carrots and red peppers contribute appetizing color as well as health-enhancing beta-carotene. Fresh herbs give you lots of no-cal, no-fat flavor, so you can cut back on fatty salad dressings.

Salads are also great ways to work lean protein into your diet. Main-dish salads in this chapter include Lean Beef with Greens and Feta, Mexican Chicken Salad, and Spicy Shrimp Salad with Cool Mango Dressing.

When dressing your salads, choose nonfat commercial mixtures, light vinaigrettes, or yogurt-based dressings such as Creamy Raspberry Dressing or Green-Herb Dressing. And remember: A salad can do much more than play second banana to your main course.

Spicy Shrimp Salad with Cool Mango Dressing

◇ *Per serving*

207 calories
2.6 g. fat
(11% of calories)
3 g. dietary fiber
153 mg. cholesterol
178 mg. sodium

1 mango
2 tablespoons lemon juice
1 pound large shrimp, peeled and deveined
1 tablespoon defatted chicken stock

1 teaspoon chili powder
¼ teaspoon hot-pepper sauce
1½ cups chopped pineapple

1 cup chopped tomatoes
1 red onion, thinly sliced
2 cups torn kale

*P*eel the mango and cut the flesh away from the pit. In a blender or food processor, puree the mango and lemon juice.

In a large nonstick frying pan over medium-high heat, combine the shrimp, stock, chili powder, and hot-pepper sauce. Stir until the shrimp are well coated with the seasonings and cooked through, about 3 minutes.

Remove from the heat. Add the pineapple, tomatoes, and onions.

Line a large platter with the kale. Spoon the salad onto the greens. Drizzle with the mango puree.

Serves 4

East Indian Rice Salad

◇ *Per serving*

194 calories
2.1 g. fat
(10% of calories)
2.9 g. dietary fiber
1 mg. cholesterol
77 mg. sodium

1 onion, minced
1 bay leaf
1 teaspoon canola oil
1 large carrot, julienned
2 cups cooked basmati rice
2 cups shredded Swiss chard
2 tablespoons raisins
3 scallions, julienned
¼ cup lemon juice
¼ teaspoon grated nutmeg
1 tablespoon grated Parmesan cheese

*I*n a large nonstick frying pan over medium heat, sauté the onions and bay leaf in the oil for 5 minutes.

Add the carrots and continue to cook until the onions are dark and fragrant and the carrots have softened, about 5 minutes.

Stir in the rice, Swiss chard, raisins, scallions, lemon juice, and nutmeg. Heat until the chard has wilted, about 2 minutes.

Remove the pan from the heat. Discard the bay leaf. Stir in the cheese.

Allow to cool to room temperature before serving.

Serves 4

◇　　　　　　　◇　　　　　　　◇

Mexican Chicken Salad

◇ *Per serving*

183 calories
4 g. fat
(20% of calories)
2.5 g. dietary fiber
66 mg. cholesterol
115 mg. sodium

½ cup lemon juice
2 jalapeño peppers, seeded and minced
2 tablespoons tomato paste
4 cloves garlic, minced
1 teaspoon dried oregano
1 teaspoon ground cumin
¼ teaspoon ground cinnamon
1 pound boneless, skinless chicken breasts
3 cups thinly sliced dark leafy greens
2 tablespoons toasted sesame seeds

*I*n a shallow glass dish, combine the lemon juice, peppers, tomato paste, garlic, oregano, cumin, and cinnamon.

Place the chicken between sheets of waxed paper or plastic wrap. Pound to an even thickness (about ⅓ to ½ inch) with a mallet. Place the chicken in the spice mixture and turn to coat all sides. Refrigerate for about 30 minutes, flipping the pieces midway.

Transfer the chicken to a lightly oiled broiler rack (reserve the marinade). Broil about 5 inches from the heat for 5 minutes per side, or until cooked through.

Place the marinade in a 1-quart saucepan. Bring to a boil and cook for about 30 seconds. Place the greens in a large bowl and pour the marinade over them. Toss to combine. Slice the chicken and serve on the greens. Sprinkle with the sesame seeds.

Serves 4

◇   ◇   ◇

POTATO AND RASPBERRY SALAD

◇ *Per serving*

130 calories
2.7 g. fat
(19% of calories)
4.4 g. dietary fiber
0 mg. cholesterol
12 mg. sodium

1 pound small potatoes	1 tablespoon raspberry vinegar	⅛ teaspoon grated nutmeg
1½ cups raspberries	1 tablespoon orange juice	
½ cup snipped chives	¼ teaspoon Dijon mustard	
2 teaspoons canola oil		

*S*team the potatoes for 8 to 10 minutes, or until easily pierced with a fork. Set aside to cool, then cut into bite-size pieces.

In a large bowl, combine the potatoes, raspberries, and chives.

In a cup, whisk together the oil, vinegar, orange juice, mustard, and nutmeg. Pour over the potatoes and toss gently.

Serves 4

APPLES AND CELERIAC WITH HONEY-MUSTARD DRESSING

2 tablespoons apple-cider vinegar
2 teaspoons coarse mustard
2 teaspoons honey
1 shallot, chopped
½ teaspoon black pepper
2 tablespoons defatted chicken stock
1 celeriac root
2 tablespoons lemon juice
2 green apples, shredded
⅔ cup nonfat yogurt
¼ cup diced red onions
2 cups shredded spinach
1 cup radish slices

*P*lace the vinegar, mustard, honey, shallots, and pepper in a blender container. Process on high speed until well mixed. With the blender running, slowly pour in the stock to form an emulsion.

Trim and wash the celeriac. Cut into a fine julienne and place in a large bowl. Add the lemon juice and combine well to keep the celeriac from discoloring. Mix in the apples, yogurt, onions, and dressing.

Serve on a bed of spinach with the radishes.

Serves 4

◇ ◇ ◇

ROTINI WITH ROSEMARY VINAIGRETTE

4 cups cooked rotini
2 cups shredded spinach
½ cup minced scallions
3 tablespoons lemon juice
1 tablespoon olive oil
1 teaspoon Dijon mustard
1 clove garlic, minced
1 teaspoon dried rosemary

0 mg. cholesterol
39 mg. sodium

*I*n a large bowl, combine the rotini, spinach, and scallions.

In a small bowl, whisk together the lemon juice, oil, mustard, garlic, and rosemary.

Pour the dressing over the rotini. Toss well to combine. Serve at room temperature or very slightly chilled.

Serves 4

◇   ◇   ◇

GARLIC AND EGGPLANT SALAD

◇ *Per serving*

308 calories
6.8 g. fat
(20% of calories)
7.5 g. dietary fiber
0 mg. cholesterol
358 mg. sodium

1 eggplant	1 tablespoon olive oil	2 cups shredded collard greens
1 whole garlic bulb	1 tablespoon dried thyme	
2 onions, thinly sliced	12 slices whole-grain bread	
2 sweet red peppers, sliced		

*P*eel the eggplant and cut into 1-inch chunks. Blanch in boiling water until just tender, about 4 minutes. Drain and pat dry.

Separate the garlic bulb into cloves and peel each.

In a 9 × 13-inch glass baking dish, combine the eggplant, garlic, onions, peppers, oil, and thyme. Stir to coat the vegetables with the oil.

Bake uncovered at 450° F until the vegetables are brown, about 25 minutes (stir a few times during cooking). Remove from the oven.

Place the bread on a baking sheet and bake until crisp, about 4 minutes per side. Cut each slice into quarters.

Serve the vegetables warm or at room temperature on a bed of collards. Eat with the bread croutons.

Serves 4

Smoked Turkey and Grapes

◇ *Per serving*

295 calories
8.3 g. fat
(25% of calories)
2 g. dietary fiber
46 mg. cholesterol
689 mg. sodium

2 tablespoons white-wine vinegar
1 teaspoon Dijon mustard
1 tablespoon olive oil
1 tablespoon minced fresh parsley
1 tablespoon snipped chives
¼ teaspoon dried chervil
¼ teaspoon dried tarragon
1 small head curly endive
12 ounces smoked turkey breast, sliced
4 cups seedless green grapes
4 slices French bread

*I*n a small bowl, whisk together the vinegar and mustard. Slowly whisk in the oil and continue until thoroughly emulsified. Stir in the parsley, chives, chervil, and tarragon.

Arrange the endive on a large platter. Top with the turkey and grapes. Drizzle with the dressing. Serve with the bread.

Serves 4

◇

Curried Potato Salad

◇ *Per serving*

180 calories
3.1 g. fat
(16% of calories)
3.5 g. dietary fiber
1 mg. cholesterol
34 mg. sodium

1 pound potatoes
¼ cup raisins
2 scallions, minced
3 tablespoons sliced almonds
½ cup nonfat yogurt
2 tablespoons chutney
1 teaspoon curry powder

*C*ut the potatoes into 1-inch chunks. Steam until tender, about 12 minutes. Transfer to a large bowl. Stir in the raisins, scallions, and almonds.

In a small bowl, whisk together the yogurt, chutney, and curry powder. Pour over the potatoes and combine well. Serve warm.

Serves 4

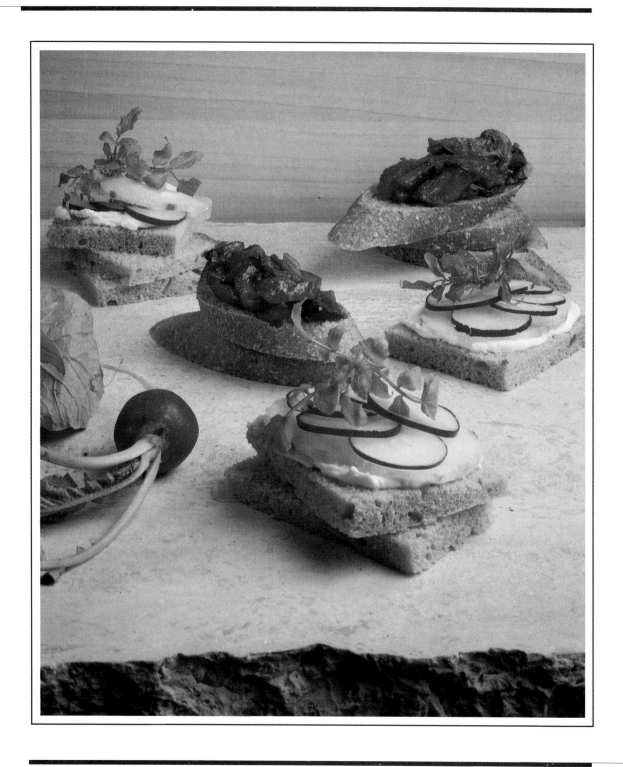

WATERCRESS CANAPÉS (PAGE 32)

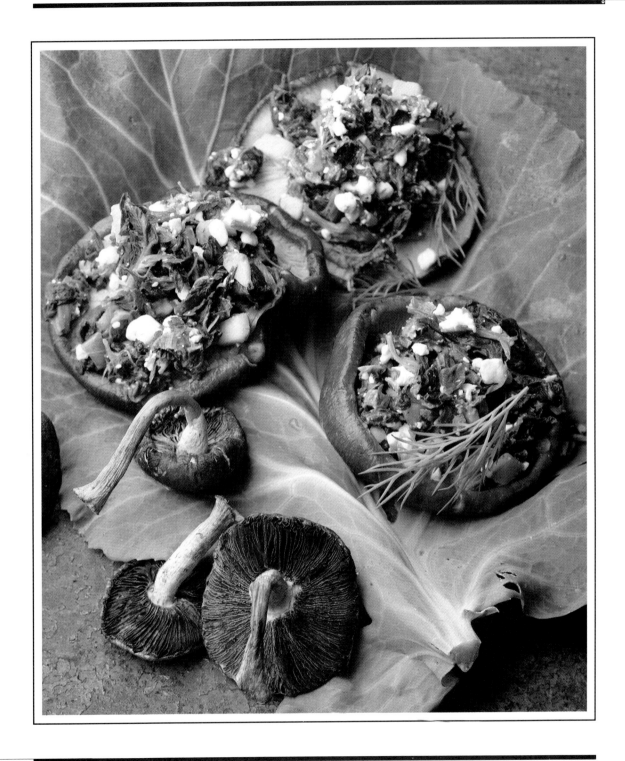

SPINACH-STUFFED MUSHROOMS (PAGE 28)

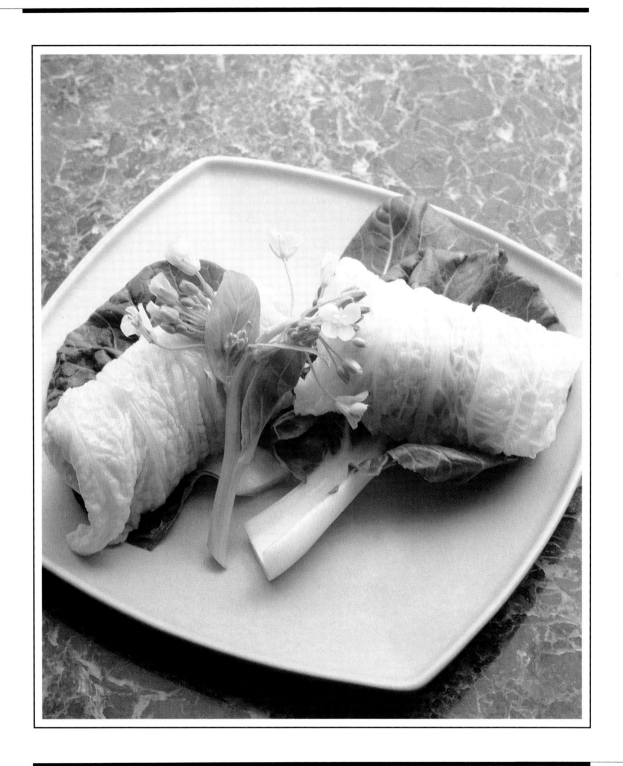

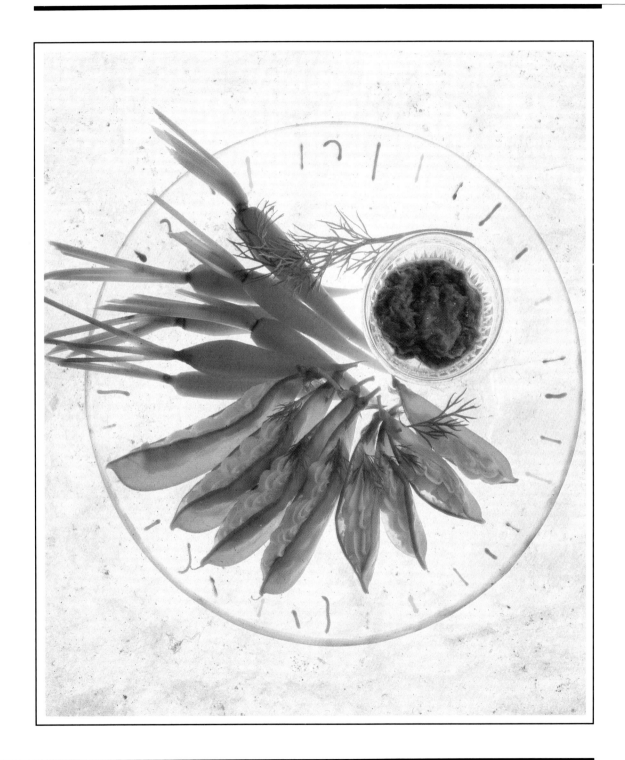

SAVORY STUFFED SNOW PEAS (PAGE 34) AND CARROT STICKS WITH DILL PESTO (PAGE 22)

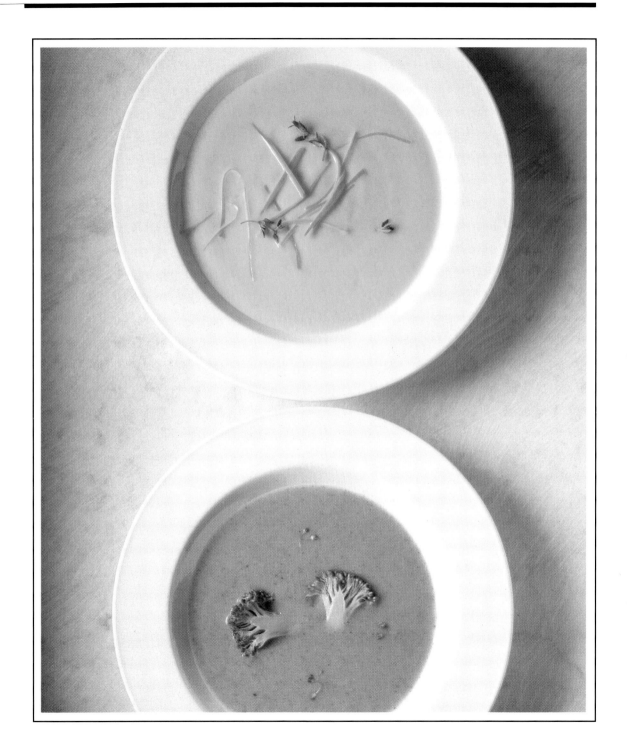

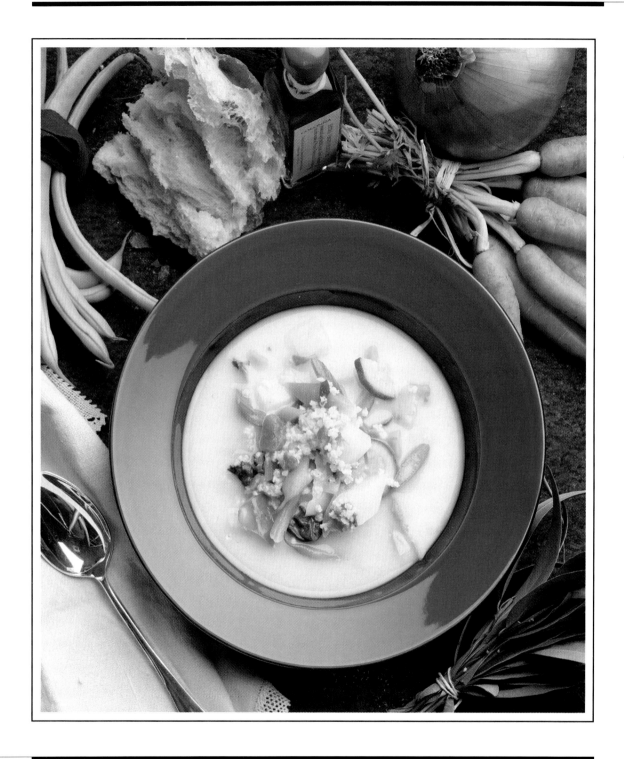

EIGHT-VEGETABLE MILLET SOUP (PAGE 49)

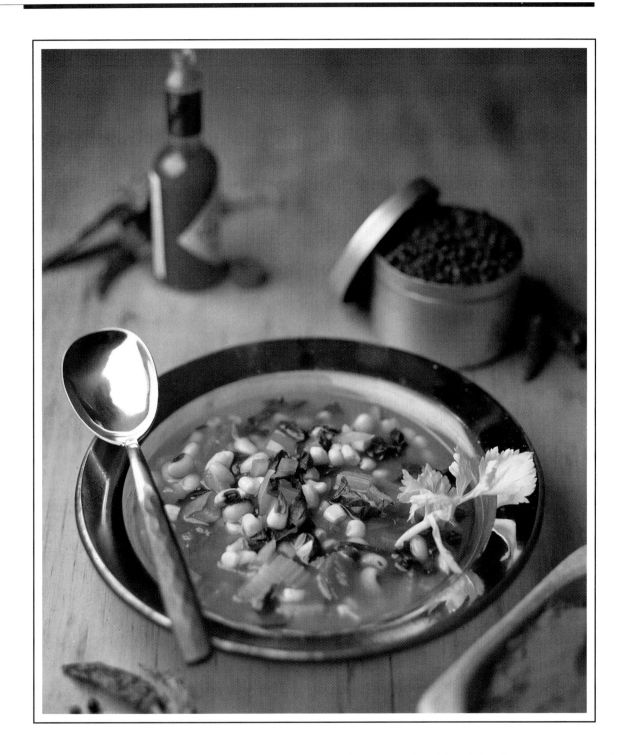

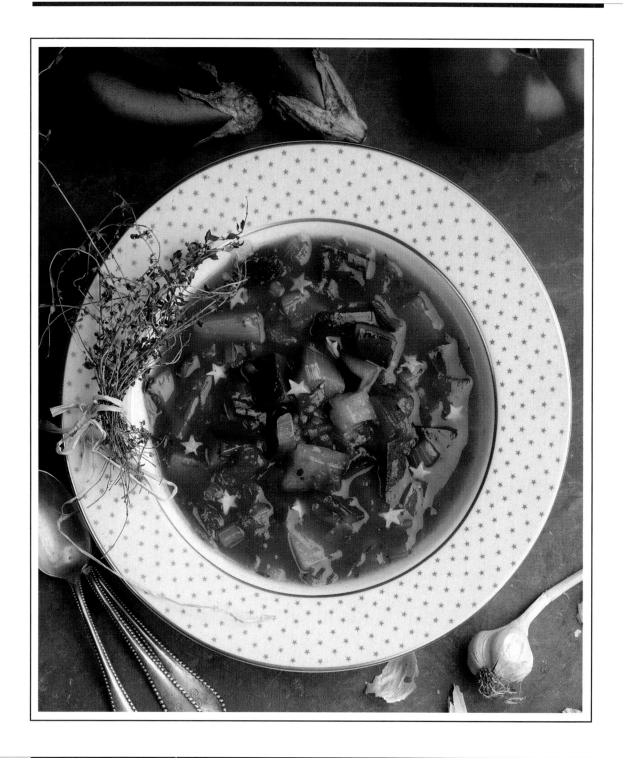

64   EGGPLANT SOUP WITH TINY PASTA (PAGE 36)

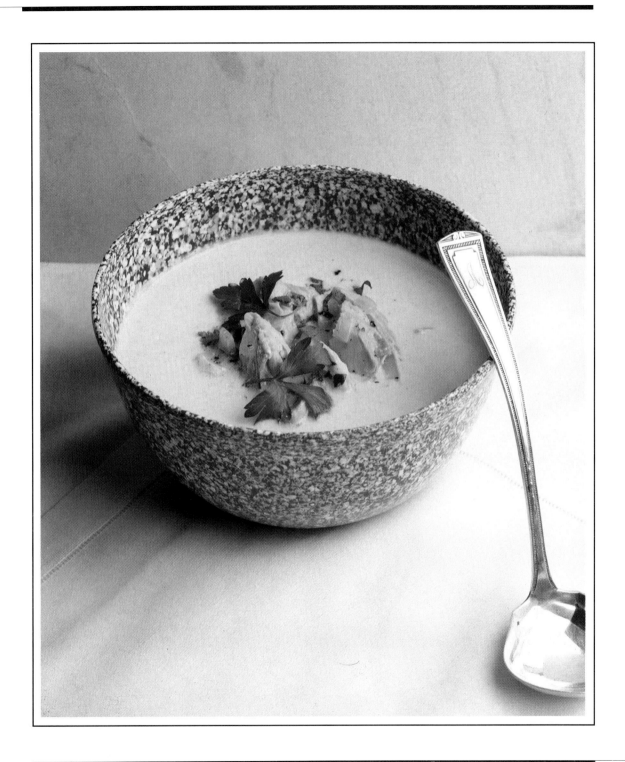

SALMON BISQUE (PAGE 47)

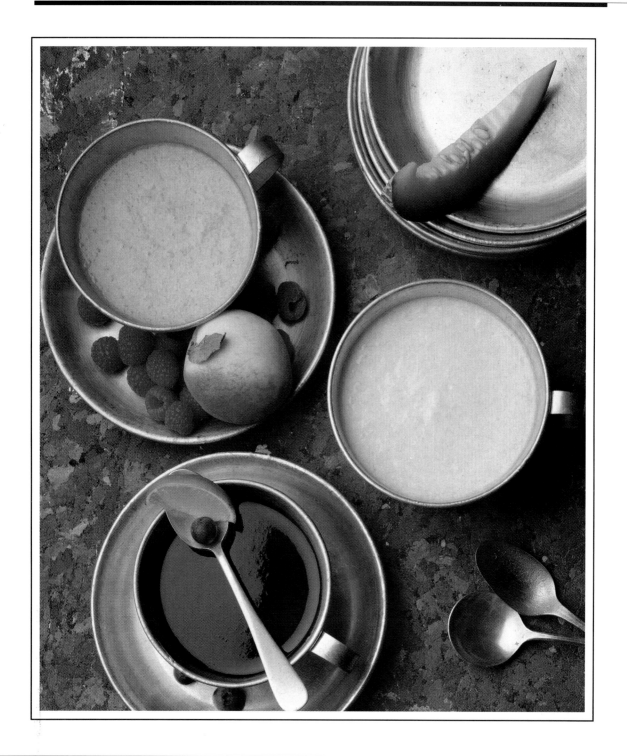

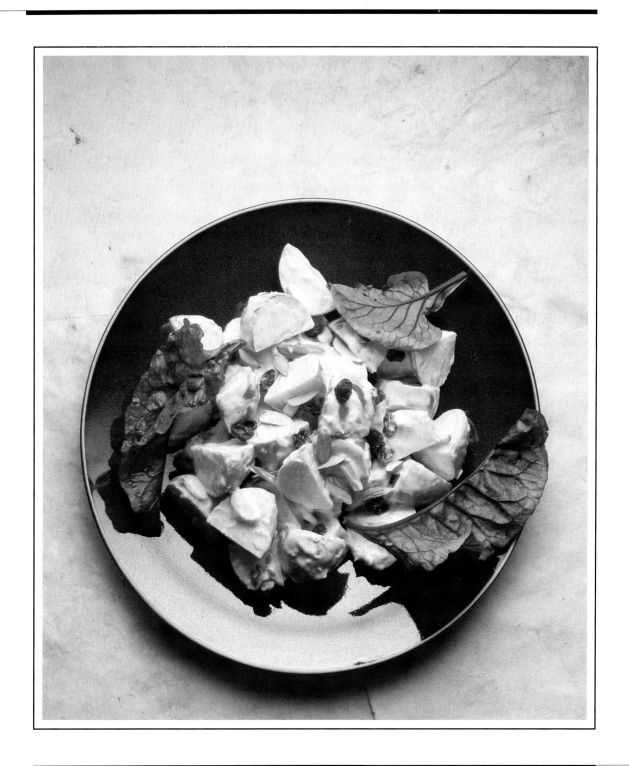

CURRIED POTATO SALAD (PAGE 56)

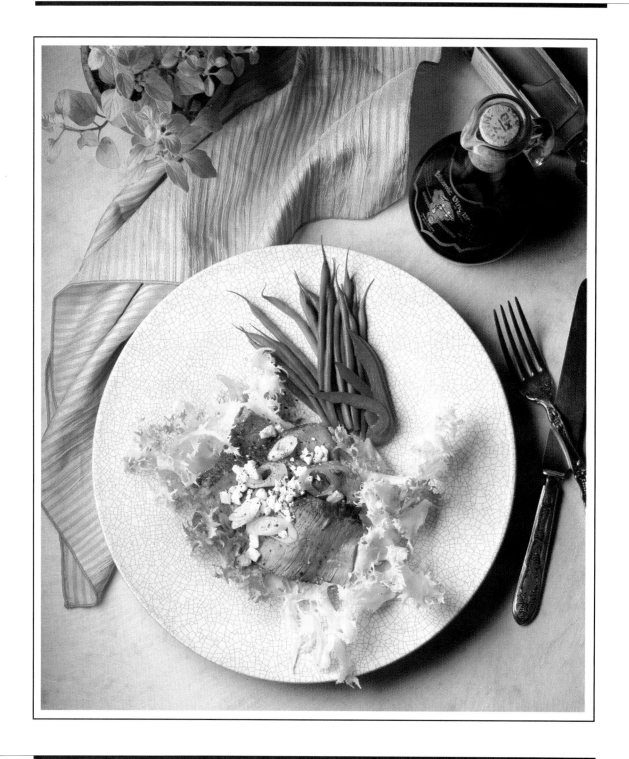

LEAN BEEF WITH GREENS AND FETA (PAGE 74)

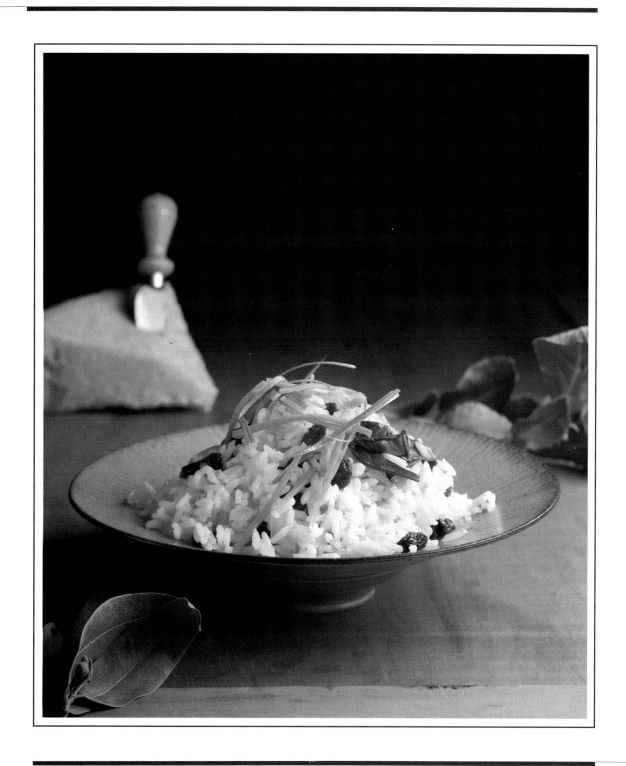

EAST INDIAN RICE SALAD (PAGE 52)

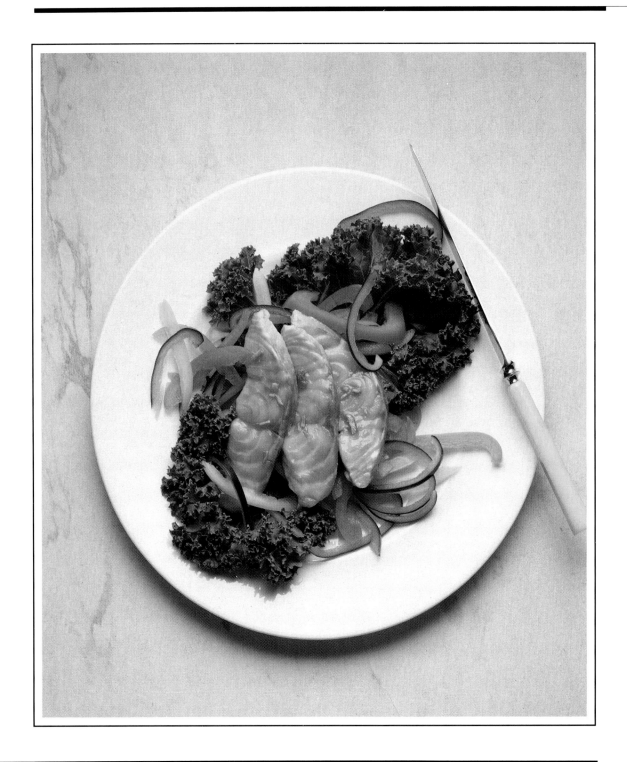

WARM SALMON SALAD (PAGE 84)

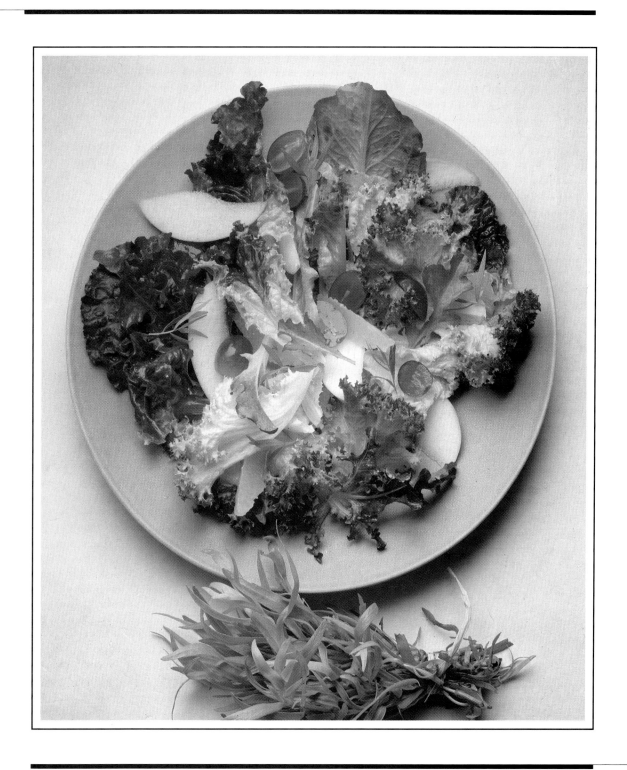

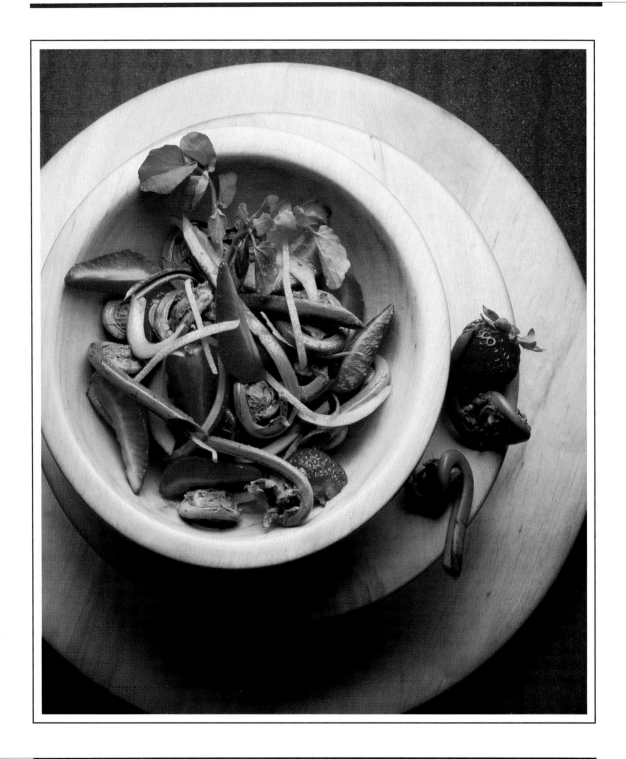

BERRIES AND GREENS (PAGE 80)

OIL'S WELL WITH OLIVE OIL

Olive oil has been highly esteemed throughout history. The Etruscans, and the Romans who succeeded them, revered it as sacred. They valued the golden oil as a healing balm and used it to massage and soothe the muscles of athletes before and after their vigorous games. In more modern times, olive oil is again regarded as a natural restorer. This monounsaturated oil shows evidence of controlling cholesterol, a major factor in heart disease.

Careful handling at home will safeguard olive oil's best qualities. Because the oil can easily pick up foreign odors and flavors, either buy it in small quantities or decant large amounts into smaller containers. Keep the bottles tightly capped or corked. Heat can cause the oil to turn rancid, so store it in a cool place. You can store large quantities in the refrigerator. Although chilling solidifies the oil, it has no effect on flavor and quality. Simply let the oil warm to room temperature for ease of pouring.

There are four major classifications of olive oil, plus another that's new.

■ *Extra-virgin* is extracted from the highest-quality, undamaged olives. This first pressing yields a green, slightly cloudy oil with a strong fruity taste. The opacity of the extra-virgin oil indicates its high quality and low acid content.

This type, which may be referred to as "fruity," is best used where its intense flavor can be appreciated without masking other flavors, such as in green salads.

■ *Virgin* oil is obtained from the second pressing of the olive paste. The olives used might not have been as ripe or unblemished. Virgin oil ranges in color from medium green to dark yellow and in flavor from lightly fruity to sweet and nutty. More economical than extra-virgin oil, virgin olive oil is also excellent for use in salad dressing and marinades.

■ *Pure* is a mixture of lower-quality virgin oil and additional oil extracted from the olive paste with an infusion of hot water. Pure olive oil is further refined, reducing the amount of acid, color, and odor present in the final product. Usually a clear gold color with only the faint oily taste of olives, it is most often used in cooking, where it adds its own subtle flavor and aroma and enhances other foods.

■ *Fine* olive oil is the last to be extracted from the olive pulp. Water and other solvents may be used to obtain this final, lower-quality extraction, which is generally not recommended for home use.

■ *Light* olive oil, the newest variety, is named not for its caloric content but for its flavor. Light is pure olive oil made with very little virgin oil. It's aimed at consumers who want to use olive oil at the stove or in salads with only a hint of the olive taste.

Bulgur and Sweet-Pepper Salad

½ cup defatted stock
½ cup bulgur
3 cloves garlic, minced
4 plum tomatoes, chopped

2 sweet red peppers, julienned
¼ cup apple-cider vinegar
2 teaspoons olive oil

½ teaspoon dried thyme
1 teaspoon snipped chives

*I*n a 1-quart saucepan, bring the stock to a boil. Add the bulgur and garlic. Cover, remove from the heat, and let stand for 20 minutes, or until the liquid has been absorbed. Fluff with a fork and place in a large bowl.

Add the tomatoes and peppers. Toss to combine.

In a cup, whisk together the vinegar, oil, thyme, and chives. Pour over the bulgur. Toss to combine.

Serves 4

◇   ◇   ◇

Lean Beef with Greens and Feta

8 ounces lean top round
1 tablespoon coarse mustard
4 cups torn chicory
2 cups sliced green beans

1 sweet red pepper, julienned
2 scallions, minced
3 tablespoons red-wine vinegar
1 teaspoon olive oil

2 tablespoons defatted beef stock
1 teaspoon dried oregano
1 tablespoon crumbled feta cheese
4 crusty rolls

*R*ub the beef on both sides with the mustard. Broil or grill about 5 inches from the heat until cooked the way you like it, about 7 minutes on each side for medium rare. Let stand for 5 minutes, then slice thinly across the grain.

In a large bowl, combine the chicory, beans, peppers, and scallions.

In a small bowl whisk together the vinegar, oil, stock, and oregano. Pour over the greens and toss to combine.

Arrange the greens on individual serving plates. Top with the beef. Sprinkle with the cheese. Serve with the rolls.

Serves 4

◇   ◇   ◇

ORANGES WITH RADISHES AND DATES

◇ *Per serving*

119 calories
1.9 g. fat
(14% of calories)
4.2 g. dietary fiber
0 mg. cholesterol
5 mg. sodium

4 large navel oranges
2 tablespoons lemon juice
1 tablespoon honey

½ teaspoon ground cinnamon
2 heads Boston lettuce
10 red radishes, thinly sliced

2 tablespoons chopped walnuts
½ cup pitted dates

*W*ith a small sharp knife, remove the peel and white pith from the oranges. Slice the oranges crosswise into ¼-inch rounds. Place on a large platter.

In a cup, whisk together the lemon juice, honey, and cinnamon. Pour over the oranges. Cover and chill for 30 minutes.

Tear the lettuce into small pieces and place in a large bowl. Add the radishes and walnuts. Drain the dressing from the oranges and pour over the lettuce. Toss well. Add the oranges and dates. Toss to combine.

Serves 6

Monkfish Salad with Tomato Chutney

◇ *Per serving*

236 calories
6.1 g. fat
(23% of calories)
3.5 g. dietary fiber
29 mg. cholesterol
89 mg. sodium

TOMATO CHUTNEY
- 3 cups chopped tomatoes
- 1 medium onion, chopped
- 1 green pepper, chopped
- ½ cup apple-cider vinegar
- 2 tablespoons honey
- 1 teaspoon ground ginger
- 1 clove garlic, minced
- 1 teaspoon mustard seeds
- ¼ teaspoon red pepper

YOGURT SAUCE
- 3 tablespoons apple-cider vinegar
- 1 teaspoon Dijon mustard
- ¾ cup nonfat yogurt
- 3 tablespoons snipped chives

SALAD
- 1 pound monkfish fillets
- 2 tablespoons lemon juice
- 1 bay leaf
- 1 tablespoon olive oil
- 2 tablespoons defatted chicken stock
- 2 tablespoons apple-cider vinegar
- 1½ cups shredded cabbage
- 1 cucumber, thinly sliced

*T*o make the tomato chutney: In a 2-quart saucepan, combine the tomatoes, onions, peppers, vinegar, honey, ginger, garlic, mustard seeds, and red pepper. Bring to a boil, then lower the heat and simmer uncovered for 1 hour, stirring frequently. Allow to cool.

To make the yogurt sauce: In a small bowl, whisk together the vinegar and mustard. Stir in the yogurt and chives. Chill until ready to use.

To make the salad: Rinse the fish in cold water. If necessary, remove any membranes. Place the fish in a large frying pan. Add the lemon juice, bay leaf, and cold water to cover.

Bring to a boil, reduce the heat to medium, cover the pan, and simmer the fish until it flakes when tested with a fork, about 8 to 10 minutes. Discard the bay leaf.

Cool slightly, then remove the fish with a slotted spoon. Separate it into large chunks, place in a large bowl, and chill for 1 hour.

the super salad bowl

In a cup, whisk together the oil, stock, and vinegar. Drizzle half over the monkfish. Toss to combine.

In a large bowl, combine the cabbage and cucumbers. Toss with the remaining dressing. Divide the mixture among serving plates. Top with the fish. Serve with the tomato chutney and the yogurt sauce.

Serves 4

◇   ◇   ◇

WILD-RICE SALAD

◇ *Per serving*

220 calories
5.8 g. fat
(24% of calories)
2.9 g. dietary fiber
2 mg. cholesterol
27 mg. sodium

4 cups water
1 cup wild rice, rinsed
2 tablespoons pine nuts
1 green pepper, julienned
1 sweet yellow pepper, julienned
2 scallions, minced

1 clove garlic, minced
1 teaspoon dried basil
½ teaspoon dried thyme
2 tablespoons red-wine vinegar
1 tablespoon lemon juice

2 teaspoons olive oil
¼ teaspoon dry mustard
1 head Boston lettuce
1 tablespoon crumbled feta cheese

*I*n a 2-quart saucepan, bring the water to a boil. Add the rice and boil uncovered for 35 minutes, or until the rice is tender but still a bit chewy. Drain well and set aside.

Heat a nonstick frying pan over medium heat. Add the pine nuts and shake the pan over heat for 2 or 3 minutes to toast the nuts. Transfer to a large bowl. Add the rice, green peppers, yellow peppers, scallions, garlic, basil, and thyme.

In a cup, whisk together the vinegar, lemon juice, oil, and mustard. Pour over the rice mixture and toss well to combine.

Serve on a bed of lettuce. Sprinkle with the cheese.

Serves 4

accent on **Health:** A Splash of Vinegar

Vinegar is one of the oldest known ingredients used in cooking. The name comes from the French words for sour wine: *vin aigre*. But vinegar is much more than fermented wine. It's a low-calorie, no-fat, sodium-free boon to salads, cooked vegetables, and even fruits.

While many varieties are made from wine—champagne, sherry, white wine, red wine, rice wine, or fruit wine—others come from ale (malt vinegar), apples (apple-cider vinegar), grains (distilled vinegar), or unfermented grapes (balsamic vinegar).

Wine vinegars vary in quality and taste. Rice-wine vinegar, for instance, is less acidic than many other types, so you can use more of it in a vinaigrette with a given amount of oil. That reduces both the grams of fat and the calories per serving.

In the town of Modena in northern Italy, a wine vinegar known as balsamic vinegar is produced. Made from special grapes that are cooked over a fire and aged in wooden casks, the vinegar is matured for years. This results in a richly colored, aromatic vinegar. Because this process is so time-consuming, balsamic and other naturally made vinegars can be expensive. But just a small amount makes a delicious difference in salads.

You can make your own flavored vinegars for home use or to give as healthful gifts. Start with plain apple-cider vinegar, white-wine vinegar, or a mixture of both. For gift giving, seek out beautiful, unusual bottles. Or simply reuse the bottle the plain vinegar came in. Remove the original label and tie a ribbon around the cap.

- *Herb vinegar.* Rinse and pat dry whole herb springs—try tarragon, thyme, rosemary, savory, basil, oregano, marjoram, or dill. Place a few sprigs in a sterile pint jar. Heat 2 cups of plain vinegar to a simmer in a small stainless steel or ceramic saucepan. Use a funnel to pour the hot vinegar into the bottle, allow to cool, and then cap tightly. Let stand for a week before using. Store at room temperature.
- *Garlic vinegar.* Skewer a peeled garlic clove and place in a sterile pint jar, alone or with herbs. Add 2 cups hot vinegar as a herb vinegar recipe, but remove the garlic after one or two days to prevent the development of botulism.
- *Berry vinegar.* Heat 2 cups of plain vinegar to a simmer as in herb vinegar recipe. Add ½ cup rinsed and dried berries, 1 tablespoon honey, and a twist of orange or lemon rind. Cool to room temperature, cover the pan, and allow to steep in a cool place for two to three days. When ready to bottle, reheat the vinegar to the simmering point, then strain into a pint jar.

the super salad bowl

Sea Kabob Salad
with Curry Vinaigrette

◇ *Per serving*

127 calories
3 g. fat
(21% of calories)
1.1 g. dietary fiber
86 mg. cholesterol
153 mg. sodium

SALAD
1/4 cup vinegar
2 cloves garlic, minced
3 bay leaves
6 ounces jumbo shrimp, peeled and deveined
6 ounces large sea scallops
6 ounces shark, cut into 1-inch chunks

3 yellow peppers, julienned

VINAIGRETTE
2 tablespoons vinegar
1 teaspoon Dijon mustard
1 teaspoon coarse mustard

1 teaspoon curry powder
2 cloves garlic, minced
1 teaspoon rinsed capers
1/4 teaspoon black pepper

*T*o make the salad: In a 9 × 13-inch baking dish, combine the vinegar, garlic, and bay leaves. Add the shrimp, scallops, and shark. Toss to coat. Cover and allow to marinate for 1 hour.

Thread the seafood onto skewers. Broil about 4 inches from the heat for 3 to 4 minutes per side. Allow to cool for a few minutes, then transfer to a large bowl. Add the peppers.

To make the vinaigrette: In a small bowl, whisk together the vinegar, Dijon mustard, coarse mustard, curry powder, garlic, capers, and pepper. Pour over the seafood mixture. Toss to coat. Serve immediately.

Serves 4

Berries and Greens

◇ *Per serving*

47 calories
1.3 g. fat
(25% of calories)
2.6 g. dietary fiber
0 mg. cholesterol
8 mg. sodium

1½ cups
watercress
leaves
1½ cups torn
arugula
1½ cups sliced
strawberries
1 red onion,
thinly sliced
½ cup
fiddlehead
ferns

2 tablespoons
apple-cider
vinegar
1 teaspoon
olive oil
¼ teaspoon
grated
orange rind

*I*n a large bowl, combine the watercress, arugula, strawberries, onions, and ferns. Sprinkle with the vinegar, oil, and orange rind. Toss to combine.

Serves 4

Asparagus and Shellfish Salad

◇ *Per serving*

99 calories
1.5 g. fat
(14% of calories)
3.1 g. dietary fiber
19 mg. cholesterol
107 mg. sodium

1 pound
asparagus
spears
¼ cup minced
shallots
¾ cup defatted
stock
1 tablespoon
vinegar

12 clams in their
shells,
scrubbed
12 mussels in
their shells,
scrubbed and
debearded
2 tablespoons
minced sweet
red peppers

2 tablespoons
minced
parsley
2 cups torn kale
1 sweet yellow
pepper, thinly
sliced

*I*n a large pot of boiling water, blanch the asparagus for 2 minutes. Drain and set aside.

In a 4-quart pot, sauté the shallots in 2 tablespoons stock for 4 minutes. Add the remaining stock and vinegar; heat to boiling. Add the clams; cover and cook for 1 minute. Add the mussels; cover and cook for 3 to 5 minutes, or until all the shells open.

Remove and discard the shells; also discard any unopened shells. Place the clams and mussels in a large bowl. Sprinkle with the red peppers and parsley.

Pour the stock liquid over the shellfish, being careful not to transfer any sediment or sand at the very bottom of the pot.

Divide the asparagus, kale, and yellow peppers among individual dinner plates. Spoon on the shellfish mixture. Serve warm or at room temperature.

Serves 4

◇   ◇   ◇

GREENS AND TANGERINES

◇ *Per serving*

77 calories
2.1 g. fat
(25% of calories)
2.2 g. dietary fiber
0 mg. cholesterol
4 mg. sodium

2 cups torn red lettuce
1½ teaspoons olive oil
2 cups tangerine sections
1 cup red grapes, halved
1 tart apple, diced
2 tablespoons lemon juice
1 teaspoon minced fresh tarragon
¼ teaspoon dried mint

*P*lace the lettuce in a large serving bowl. Toss with the oil until coated.

Add the tangerines, grapes, and apples. Sprinkle with the lemon juice, tarragon, and mint. Toss to combine.

Serves 4

accent on Health: Dress for Success

Salad dressing can make or break a salad, especially one composed largely of health-rendering greens and vegetables. The right dressing enhances the flavor of the basic ingredients without overwhelming them or undermining their health qualities. The wrong dressing can smother a nutritious food under a blanket of fat and calories. Here are some ways to dress a salad that make good sense.

Remember that no matter what type of dressing you choose, you should use only enough to lightly coat the salad. One way to do that is to mix your salad in an oversized bowl, large enough to toss the ingredients freely and to thoroughly distribute a modest amount of dressing. To add more flavor to your salad, rub the inside of the bowl with a cut clove of garlic before adding the salad.

◇ ───────────────────────────

Green-Herb Dressing

1 cup low-fat cottage cheese	1 tablespoon honey
1 cup nonfat yogurt	2 teaspoons Dijon mustard
3 tablespoons grated Sapsago or Parmesan cheese	2 teaspoons minced shallots
2 tablespoons lemon juice	1 teaspoon dried basil
	¼ teaspoon black pepper

In a blender or food processor, process the cottage cheese until very smooth. Transfer to a medium bowl.

Whisk in the yogurt, Sapsago or Parmesan, lemon juice, honey, mustard, shallots, basil, and pepper.

Makes about 2½ cups

◇ *Per tablespoon:* *12 calories, 0.2 g. fat (15% of calories), <0.1 g. dietary fiber, <1 mg. cholesterol, 40 mg. sodium*

Watercress Dressing

½ cup nonfat yogurt

½ cup packed watercress leaves

2 tablespoons vinegar

2 scallions, thinly sliced

1 clove garlic, minced

½ teaspoon dried tarragon

In a blender, combine the yogurt, watercress, vinegar, scallions, garlic, and tarragon. Process until smooth.

Makes 1 cup

◇ *Per tablespoon:* 5 calories, <1 g. fat (4% of calories), <0.1 g. dietary fiber, 0 mg. cholesterol, 6 mg. sodium

◇ ————————————————

Creamy Raspberry Dressing

1 cup nonfat yogurt

1 cup raspberries

¼ teaspoon grated orange rind

¼ teaspoon grated lime rind

¼ teaspoon dried basil

Line a strainer with cheesecloth. Add the yogurt and allow to drain over a bowl for 30 minutes. Transfer to a medium bowl.

Puree the raspberries in a food processor. Fold into the yogurt. Add the orange rind, lime rind, and basil. Combine well.

Makes 1 cup

◇ *Per tablespoon:* 12 calories, 0.1 g. fat (8% of calories), 0.3 g. dietary fiber, <1 mg. cholesterol, 11 mg. sodium

WARM SALMON SALAD

◇ *Per serving*

225 calories
5.5 g. fat
(22% of calories)
0.6 g. dietary fiber
16 mg. cholesterol
541 mg. sodium

2 tablespoons low-sodium soy sauce
2 teaspoons peeled minced gingerroot
1 teaspoon honey
2 cloves garlic, minced
⅛ teaspoon red pepper

4 ounces salmon fillet
1½ teaspoons olive oil
2 tablespoons balsamic vinegar
2 tablespoons minced shallots
1 tablespoon lemon juice

1 pound kale, torn into bite-size pieces
2 green peppers, julienned
⅓ cup defatted stock
4 slices French bread

*I*n a 9 × 13-inch baking dish, whisk together the soy sauce, ginger, honey, garlic, and red pepper.

Cutting on the bias, slice the salmon into thin pieces. Add to the soy mixture, turning to coat each piece on both sides. Let stand about 15 minutes.

In a small bowl, whisk together the oil, vinegar, shallots, and lemon juice.

Divide the kale among salad plates. Top with the peppers.

In a large nonstick frying pan over medium-high heat, heat the stock. Add the salmon and cook about 10 to 15 seconds per side. Add to the salad plates. Drizzle with the oil and vinegar dressing. Serve warm with the bread.

Serves 4

the super salad bowl

CHAPTER FIVE ◇

Breads and Breakfasts

*B*reads, muffins, scones, waffles, pancakes—all this and more can be yours from a healthy bakery. Made with high-fiber, low-fat grains, these goodies are a smart choice for just about anybody, from weight watchers and the cholesterol conscious to those with diabetes or high blood pressure. Many of these treats get sweetness from added fruit or a savory tang from vegetables and herbs. Both types serve as a gentle reminder that baked goods can greatly enhance a nutritious diet.

If yeast bread is your passion, you'll love Dilled Carrot Bread and Pineapple Focaccia, a variation on a traditional Italian flat bread. When time is at a premium, opt for muffins or quick breads. One-Hour Oat Bread has lots of cholesterol-lowering oats and oat bran, plus raisins for a hint of sweetness. Cranberry Bread is a welcome treat all year around (freeze some cranberries for summer enjoyment). As for muffins, we've got a basketful, including pecan-oat, cornmeal-cheese, prune, carrot, and cranberry.

Don't forget that batter-based pancakes and waffles can also be low-fat breakfast, brunch, and dessert fare. Egg whites or egg substitute keeps cholesterol low, and canola or olive oil adds beneficial monounsaturates to a heart-smart diet. Serve these special goodies with plenty of fresh fruit or high-fiber "preserves," such as Carrot Spread, Prune Butter, or Savory Pear Spread. You'll relish their natural sweetness.

APPLE BREAKFAST BREAD

◇ *Per slice*

167 calories
3.7 g. fat
(20% of calories)
3.6 g. dietary fiber
<1 mg. cholesterol
124 mg. sodium

2 apples
1 cup whole wheat flour
1 cup unbleached flour
½ cup oat bran
1 teaspoon baking powder
1 teaspoon baking soda
1 teaspoon ground cinnamon
⅓ cup coarsely chopped almonds
3 egg whites
¾ cup nonfat yogurt
⅓ cup maple syrup
1 tablespoon canola oil
1 teaspoon vanilla extract
¼ cup apricot all-fruit preserves
1 tablespoon orange juice

Coat a 9-inch tube pan with nonstick spray.

Cut 1 apple into slices and arrange them around the bottom of the pan. Chop the other apple and set aside.

In a large bowl, mix the whole wheat flour, unbleached flour, oat bran, baking powder, baking soda, and cinnamon. Stir in the chopped apples and almonds.

In a medium bowl, combine the egg whites, yogurt, maple syrup, oil, and vanilla.

Pour the liquid ingredients over the flour mixture. Stir to combine, but don't overmix.

Add the batter to the prepared pan and level out the top. Bake at 375°F for 25 minutes.

Let cool for 5 minutes on a wire rack. Run a knife between the bread and the sides of the pan to loosen the bread. Let stand for 10 minutes before unmolding. Cool completely before serving.

Combine the preserves and orange juice in a 1-quart saucepan. Heat briefly to melt the preserves. Drizzle over the bread.

Makes 1 loaf; 12 slices

PINEAPPLE FOCACCIA

½ cup warm
   water (110° F)
1 tablespoon
   active dry
   yeast
2 teaspoons
   honey

1 tablespoon
   canola oil
1 cup
   unbleached
   flour
½ cup whole
   wheat flour

¾ cup dried
   pineapple,
   thinly sliced
2 tablespoons
   sesame seeds

*I*n a large bowl, mix the water, yeast, honey, and 2 teaspoons of the oil. Let stand for about 2 minutes, or until the yeast is dissolved.

Sift together the unbleached flour and whole wheat flour. Add to the yeast mixture. Stir well.

Turn the dough out onto a floured surface and knead until elastic, about 5 or 6 minutes. Let stand 5 minutes.

Coat two 9-inch round cake pans with nonstick spray. Roll the dough into two circles and place in the pans. Divide the pineapple between the pans and press it into the dough. Brush lightly with the remaining oil. Sprinkle with the sesame seeds.

Bake at 500° F for 7 minutes. Cover with foil to prevent the fruit from burning. Bake another 5 to 8 minutes.

Remove from the pans and cut with kitchen shears or a pizza cutter. Serve warm.

Serves 4

Sweet Potato Scones

◇ *Per scone*

48 calories
1.3 g. fat
(24% of calories)
0.9 g. dietary fiber
<1 mg. cholesterol
42 mg. sodium

½ cup whole
  wheat flour
½ cup
  unbleached
  flour
¼ cup corn bran
1 teaspoon
  cream of
  tartar
½ teaspoon
  baking soda

⅛ teaspoon
  ground
  cinnamon
⅛ teaspoon
  grated nutmeg
¾ cup shredded
  sweet
  potatoes

¼ cup raisins,
  chopped
⅓ cup buttermilk
1½ tablespoons
  canola oil

*I*n a large bowl, mix the whole wheat flour, unbleached flour, corn bran, cream of tartar, baking soda, cinnamon, and nutmeg. Stir in the sweet potatoes and raisins.

Add the buttermilk and oil. With floured hands, knead the mixture for about 2 minutes.

On a lightly floured surface, roll out the dough to a generous ¼ inch thick. Cut out 2½-inch rounds. Transfer to a lightly oiled baking sheet. Use all the dough by rerolling leftovers.

Bake at 475° F for 6 to 8 minutes. Serve warm.

Makes about 18

Cornmeal-Cheese Muffins

◇ *Per muffin*

129 calories
3.6 g. fat
(25% of calories)
3.1 g. dietary fiber

1½ cups
  cornmeal
½ cup whole
  wheat flour
2½ teaspoons
  baking
  powder

¾ cup skim milk
¼ cup egg
  substitute
2 tablespoons
  olive oil
2 tablespoons
  honey

1 cup corn
¼ cup shredded
  low-fat
  Monterey
  Jack cheese

*I*n a large bowl, combine the cornmeal, flour, and baking powder.

In a medium bowl, combine the milk, egg substitute, oil, and honey.

Stir the liquid ingredients into the dry ingredients until just blended, but don't overmix. Fold in the corn and cheese.

Coat 12 muffin cups with nonstick spray. Fill about three-quarters full with the batter. Bake at 375°F for 15 minutes.

Makes 12

◇   ◇   ◇

ONE-HOUR OAT BREAD

◇ *Per slice*

209 calories
2.6 g. fat
(11% of calories)
6.1 g. dietary fiber
2 mg. cholesterol
191 mg. sodium

2 cups whole wheat flour
1 cup oat bran
1 cup rolled oats
¼ cup raisins
1 tablespoon baking powder
2 cups buttermilk

*I*n a large bowl, combine the flour, oat bran, oats, raisins, and baking powder.

Pour in the buttermilk and use a large rubber spatula to combine well. If the dough becomes too stiff to stir, flour your hands and finish mixing by hand.

Shape the dough into a round loaf 7 inches in diameter. Smooth the top and sides.

Line a baking sheet with parchment paper and set the loaf on it. Use a sharp knife to slash an X about ¼ inch deep in the top. If any raisins are visible, poke them into the dough with your finger so they won't burn.

Sprinkle the loaf with a bit of flour. Bake at 425°F for about 45 minutes, or until the bottom of the loaf sounds hollow when tapped.

Let cool completely before slicing.

Makes 1 loaf; 8 slices

accent on Health: High-Fiber Spreads

Keep your whole-grain breads, muffins, and scones naturally healthy with fiber-rich spreads instead of high-fat butter. Here are three fiber champs.

◇ ———————————————————

Carrot Spread

2 cups shredded
carrots

2 cups apple
juice

2 tablespoons
honey

2 tablespoons
lemon juice

1 tablespoon
grated lemon
rind

In a 2-quart saucepan, combine the carrots, apple juice, honey, lemon juice, and lemon rind. Simmer over medium heat, stirring frequently, until thick, about 30 to 45 minutes.
Store in a tightly closed container in the refrigerator.

Makes about 1½ cups

◇ *Per tablespoon:* *20 calories, <0.1 g. fat (2% of calories), 0.3 g. dietary fiber, 0 mg. cholesterol, 4 mg. sodium*

◇ ———————————————————

Prune Butter

2 cups pitted
prunes

1¾ cups apple
juice

8 dried figs,
stems removed

1 teaspoon
vanilla extract

1 teaspoon
grated orange
rind

In a 2-quart saucepan, combine the prunes, apple juice, figs, vanilla, and orange rind. Bring to a simmer and cook over low heat, stirring frequently, for 30 minutes.

Let the mixture cool slightly. Transfer to a food processor or blender. Process until smooth (if mixture becomes too thick, thin with additional apple juice).

Store in a tightly closed container in the refrigerator.

Makes about 2 cups

◇ *Per tablespoon:* *34 calories, 0.1 g. fat (3% of calories), 1 g. dietary fiber, 0 mg. cholesterol, 1 mg. sodium*

◇ ───────────────────────────────

Savory Pear Spread

5 ripe pears, chopped	1 tablespoon apple-cider vinegar
2 tablespoons lemon juice	½ teaspoon ground cinnamon
2 tablespoons honey	¼ teaspoon ground allspice
1 tablespoon peeled grated gingerroot	¼ teaspoon grated nutmeg

In a 2-quart saucepan, combine the pears, lemon juice, honey, ginger, vinegar, cinnamon, allspice, and nutmeg. Cook over low heat for 30 to 40 minutes, or until the pears are very tender.

In a food processor or blender, process the mixture until chunky. If the mixture is not thick, return it to the saucepan and stir over medium heat until desired thickness is reached.

Store in a tightly closed container in the refrigerator.

Makes about 2 cups

◇ *Per tablespoon:* *20 calories, 0.1 g. fat (5% of calories), 0.7 g. dietary fiber, 0 mg. cholesterol, 0 mg. sodium*

FRUIT BREAD

◇ *Per slice*

142 calories
4 g. fat
(25% of calories)
2.6 g. dietary fiber
<1 mg. cholesterol
139 mg. sodium

2 cups thinly
   sliced carrots
1 cup buttermilk
½ cup egg
   substitute
⅓ cup canola oil
⅓ cup honey
2 cups whole
   wheat flour

1 cup
   unbleached
   flour
2 teaspoons
   baking soda
1 teaspoon
   baking
   powder

½ teaspoon
   ground ginger
½ teaspoon
   grated nutmeg
1 cup chopped
   apricots
⅔ cup chopped
   pitted dates

*P*lace the carrots in a 1-quart saucepan. Add cold water to cover. Bring to a boil and cook until the carrots are tender, about 15 minutes. Drain and puree in a food mill or food processor. Measure out 1¼ cups of puree and place in a large bowl. (Reserve any remaining puree for another use.)

Add the buttermilk, egg substitute, oil, and honey. Combine well.

Sift together the whole wheat flour, unbleached flour, baking soda, baking powder, ginger, and nutmeg. Stir into the carrot mixture.

Fold in the apricots and dates.

Coat two 8½ × 4½-inch loaf pans with nonstick spray and lightly flour them. Divide the dough between the pans.

Bake at 350° F for 45 to 60 minutes, or until a tester inserted in the center comes out clean. Cool in the pans 10 minutes. Then remove and cool on wire racks before slicing.

Makes 2 loaves; 24 slices

ORANGE MUFFINS

◇ *Per muffin*

126 calories
2.6 g. fat
(19% of calories)
3.3 g. dietary fiber

1½ cups whole
   wheat flour
½ cup bran
½ cup raisins
1½ teaspoons
   baking soda

¾ cup orange
   juice
¼ cup egg
   substitute
¼ cup honey

2 tablespoons
   canola oil
Grated rind of 1
   orange

0 mg. cholesterol
115 mg. sodium

*I*n a large bowl, combine the flour, bran, raisins, and baking soda.

In a medium bowl, mix the orange juice, egg substitute, honey, oil, and orange rind.

Stir the liquid ingredients into the dry ingredients until just blended, but don't overmix.

Coat 12 muffin cups with nonstick spray. Fill about three-quarters full with the batter. Bake at 375°F for 15 minutes.

Makes 12

◇   ◇   ◇

CINNAMON-SCENTED FRENCH TOAST

◇ *Per serving*

238 calories
5.4 g. fat
(20% of calories)
5.1 g. dietary fiber
1 mg. cholesterol
280 mg. sodium

½ cup evaporated skim milk
2 egg whites
⅛ teaspoon ground cinnamon
⅛ teaspoon grated nutmeg

8 slices whole wheat or whole-grain bread
1 tablespoon canola oil

3 peaches, sliced
1 cup raspberries

*I*n a small bowl, whisk together the milk, egg whites, cinnamon, and nutmeg. Pour into a 9 × 13-inch baking dish.

Cut the bread in half for easier handling. Briefly soak the bread in the milk mixture, flipping the pieces to coat both sides.

Coat a large nonstick frying pan with nonstick spray. Heat the pan over medium-high heat. Pour in half of the oil. Add half of the bread and brown the pieces on both sides, about 2½ minutes per side.

Repeat with the remaining oil and bread. Serve warm, topped with the peaches and raspberries.

Serves 4

CRANBERRY MUFFINS

1 ⅓ cups whole wheat flour
⅓ cup wheat germ
1 tablespoon baking powder
¾ cup skim milk
⅓ cup honey
¼ cup egg substitute
2 tablespoons canola oil
1 cup coarsely chopped cranberries

*I*n a large bowl, combine the flour, wheat germ, and baking powder.

In a medium bowl, combine the milk, honey, egg substitute, and oil.

Stir the liquid ingredients into the dry ingredients until just blended, but don't overmix. Fold in the cranberries.

Coat 12 muffin cups with nonstick spray. Fill about three-quarters full with batter. Bake at 375°F for 20 to 25 minutes.

Makes 12

PECAN-OAT MUFFINS

1 cup oat bran
⅔ cup rolled oats
⅓ cup whole wheat flour
⅓ cup unbleached flour
¼ cup chopped pecans
3 tablespoons raisins
1 tablespoon baking powder
¼ cup egg substitute
1 ¼ cups buttermilk
¼ cup maple syrup
2 teaspoons canola oil
1 ½ teaspoons vanilla extract

*I*n a large bowl, mix the oat bran, oats, whole wheat flour, unbleached flour, pecans, raisins, and baking powder.

In a medium bowl, whisk together the egg substitute, buttermilk, maple syrup, oil, and vanilla.

Pour the liquid ingredients over the dry ingredients. Mix until just combined, about 10 or 15 strokes, but don't overmix.

Lightly coat 12 muffin cups with nonstick spray. Spoon the batter into the cups. Bake at 400°F for about 20 minutes, or until the tops are lightly golden and rounded.

Makes 12

◇   ◇   ◇

RISE AND SHINE

The success of yeast-risen breads and rolls depends, quite logically, on yeast. The single-celled fungi that make up yeast convert starches in dough into carbon dioxide, which inflates the dough into a nice plump bread shape. If you're confused about the various types of yeast available, here's a short primer:

■ *Active dry yeast* is the most commonly used form. This granular yeast comes in individual packets or bulk form. Kept under refrigeration, it lasts for months. (It's said that dry yeast found in Egyptian tombs was still viable after centuries.) But for best results, heed the expiration date on the package. If using bulk yeast, transfer it to a jar with a tight-fitting lid and mark the date on the jar. If the yeast is more than a year old, proof it before using. Use 2½ to 3 teaspoons of bulk yeast to equal one individual packet.

■ *Rapid-rise yeast* is a type of dry yeast that allows bread to rise much faster than regular yeast. It comes in individual packets.

■ *Compressed cake yeast* comes in little foil-wrapped blocks. A ⅔-ounce cake equals one packet of dry yeast. When fresh, compressed yeast is crumbly and falls apart easily. It is much more perishable than dry yeast and stays fresh for only two weeks under refrigeration. For longer storage, you may freeze the yeast. Wrap it tightly, then freeze it in a container filled with flour. The flour insulation helps the yeast to freeze slowly. It keeps for three to six months. Thaw at room temperature.

CARAWAY PANCAKES

◇ *Per serving*

320 calories
1 g. fat
(3% of calories)
5 g. dietary fiber
3 mg. cholesterol
198 mg. sodium

PANCAKES
½ cup whole
   wheat flour
½ cup
   unbleached
   flour
1 teaspoon
   baking
   powder
½ teaspoon
   ground
   caraway
   seeds
½ teaspoon
   ground
   cinnamon
⅓ cup golden
   raisins
1 apple, minced
½ cup buttermilk
½ cup nonfat
   yogurt
¼ cup egg
   substitute
2 tablespoons
   maple syrup

TOPPING
2 cups chunky
   applesauce
1 cup nonfat
   vanilla yogurt
¼ teaspoon
   ground
   cinnamon

*T*o make the pancakes: In a medium bowl, sift together the whole wheat flour, unbleached flour, baking powder, caraway, and cinnamon. Stir in the raisins and apples.

In a small bowl, combine the buttermilk, yogurt, egg substitute, and maple syrup.

Pour the liquid ingredients into the dry ingredients. Stir to combine.

Coat a nonstick frying pan with nonstick spray. Heat on medium-high. Drop tablespoon-size mounds of batter into the pan. Cook 2 to 3 minutes, then flip and continue cooking until richly browned and puffed.

To make the topping: In a small bowl, mix the applesauce, yogurt, and cinnamon. Serve over the pancakes.

Serves 4

POTATO WAFFLES WITH PEACH SAUCE

◇ *Per serving*

410 calories
10.9 g. fat
(24% of calories)
4.2 g. dietary fiber
4 mg. cholesterol
580 mg. sodium

WAFFLES
½ cup whole
   wheat flour
½ cup
   unbleached
   flour
2 teaspoons
   baking
   powder
¼ teaspoon
   ground
   allspice

1 cup skim milk
½ cup egg
   substitute
1 tablespoon
   honey
1 tablespoon
   canola oil
2 cups mashed
   potatoes
¼ cup chopped
   hazelnuts
3 egg whites

PEACH SAUCE
1¼ cups nonfat
   yogurt
2 peaches,
   chopped
2 tablespoons
   maple syrup
⅛ teaspoon
   grated
   nutmeg

*T*o *make the waffles:* Sift the whole wheat flour, unbleached flour, baking powder, and allspice into a large bowl.

In a medium bowl, combine the milk, egg substitute, honey, and oil. Stir in the potatoes and hazelnuts.

Pour the liquid ingredients into the dry ingredients and mix well.

In a clean bowl with clean beaters, beat the egg whites until stiff. Fold into the batter.

Heat a waffle iron and lightly brush the grids with oil. Pour in enough batter to just fill. Close and cook until the steaming stops and the waffles are crisp. (Because of the moisture in the potatoes, these waffles will take longer to bake than other waffles.)

To make the peach sauce: In a small bowl, combine the yogurt, peaches, maple syrup, and nutmeg. Serve over the waffles.

Serves 4

MICRO METHOD: Raising Yeast Bread

Made traditionally, yeast breads take hours to rise in the legendary "warm place." That's fine if you're not in a hurry and have time to hang around the house. But when time or patience is in short supply, you can get an assist from your microwave. The only catch: You need a full-size microwave with multipower settings.

Here's how to tell if your particular oven is suitable for the task.

- Place 2 tablespoons of cold stick margarine in a small cup. Position the cup in the center of the oven.
- Select 10 percent power (low) and run the microwave for 4 minutes. If the margarine melts completely, your microwave is unsuitable to raise yeast breads.

To raise yeast bread:

- Shape the dough into a ball and place in a lightly oiled bowl. Turn the dough to coat all sides with the oil.
- Cover the bowl loosely with waxed paper. Set aside.
- Fill a 4-cup glass measuring cup with 3 cups of water. Heat the water on full power for 6 to 8 minutes, or until boiling.
- Add the bowl of dough to the microwave next to the water.
- Run the microwave on low (10 percent) for about 15 minutes, or until the dough has doubled in size.
- Punch the dough down and divide it in half. Cover, let rest 10 minutes, then shape each half into a loaf.
- Place each loaf in a lightly oiled $8\frac{1}{2} \times 4\frac{1}{2}$-inch ceramic or glass loaf pan. Set aside.
- Again heat the 3 cups of water until boiling (about 4 to 5 minutes this time).
- Add the loaf pans to the microwave beside the water. Cover loosely with waxed paper.
- Heat on low (10 percent) for about 7 minutes, or until the dough nearly doubles in size.
- Bake the dough in a conventional oven according to your recipe.

DILLED CARROT BREAD

◇ *Per slice*

107 calories
1.7 g. fat
(14% of calories)
2.3 g. dietary fiber
2 mg. cholesterol
39 mg. sodium

¼ cup lukewarm water
2 teaspoons honey
1 tablespoon active dry yeast
1¼ cups shredded carrots
¾ cup dry-curd cottage cheese

¼ cup egg substitute
¼ cup grated Parmesan cheese
1 tablespoon olive oil
1 teaspoon dill seeds
½ teaspoon caraway seeds

½ teaspoon salt (optional)
1¾ cups whole wheat flour
1¼ cups unbleached flour

*I*n a large bowl, combine the water and honey. Sprinkle on the yeast and stir to combine. Set aside for 10 minutes to proof (the yeast will become foamy).

Add the carrots, cottage cheese, egg substitute, Parmesan, oil, dill, caraway, and salt (if used).

Stir in the whole wheat flour, using a wooden spoon. Add enough of the unbleached flour to form a sticky dough that comes away from the sides of the bowl.

Coat a large bowl with nonstick spray. Add the dough and turn to coat all sides. Cover with plastic wrap and towels. Place in a warm, draft-free spot and let rise until doubled in bulk, about 1 hour.

Stir down the dough with an oiled spoon.

Coat a 9 × 5-inch loaf pan or 1½-quart casserole dish with nonstick spray. Flour your hands lightly, transfer the dough to the pan, and pat it in evenly. Cover with a towel. Let rise in a warm place until doubled in bulk, about 45 minutes.

Bake at 375°F for 40 to 45 minutes, or until the bread sounds hollow when tapped.

Cool in the pan for 10 minutes. Turn out onto a wire rack. Cool completely before slicing.

Makes 1 loaf; 16 slices

POTATO-CHEESE BREAD

◇ *Per slice*

127 calories
2 g. fat
(14% of calories)
2.4 g. dietary fiber
<1 mg. cholesterol
45 mg. sodium

2¼ cups defatted chicken stock
⅓ cup grated Sapsago or Parmesan cheese
2 tablespoons olive oil
2 tablespoons honey

1 teaspoon dried thyme
1 teaspoon dillweed
2 tablespoons active dry yeast

1½ cups mashed potatoes
2¾ cups whole wheat flour
2¾ cups unbleached flour

*I*n a 3-quart saucepan, heat the stock to lukewarm. Remove from the heat. Add the cheese, oil, honey, thyme, and dill. Gently stir in the yeast. Stir in the mashed potatoes. Set aside for 10 minutes to proof (the yeast will become foamy).

In a large bowl, mix the whole wheat flour and unbleached flour. Gradually stir 4 cups of flour into the potato mixture.

Turn the dough onto a floured surface and knead in the remaining flour. Knead for about 10 minutes, or until the dough is smooth and elastic.

Lightly oil a large bowl. Add the dough and turn to coat all sides. Allow to rise in a warm, draft-free place for 30 to 40 minutes, or until doubled in bulk.

Punch down the dough and knead for 1 minute. Divide into two portions and form into loaves.

Coat two 8½ × 4½-inch loaf pans with nonstick spray. Add the dough, cover, and let rise for 30 minutes, or until doubled in bulk.

Bake at 350°F for 30 to 35 minutes, or until the loaves sound hollow when tapped.

Allow the loaves to cool on wire racks for 30 minutes.

Makes 2 loaves; 12 slices

PECAN WAFFLES WITH STRAWBERRY SAUCE

◇ *Per serving*

371 calories
10.1 g. fat
(25% of calories)
6.9 g. dietary fiber
0 mg. cholesterol
171 mg. sodium

WAFFLES
- ¾ cup whole wheat flour
- ¾ cup unbleached flour
- 1½ teaspoons baking powder
- ½ cup chopped pecans
- 1¼ cups apricot nectar
- ½ cup egg substitute
- ¼ cup maple syrup

SAUCE
- 2 cups sliced strawberries
- ½ cup apricot nectar
- 2 tablespoons maple syrup

To make the waffles: In a large bowl, sift together the whole wheat flour, unbleached flour, and baking powder. Stir in the pecans.

In a medium bowl, whisk together the nectar, egg substitute, and maple syrup.

Pour the liquid ingredients over the flour mixture. Stir to combine, but don't overmix.

Heat a waffle iron, and lightly brush the grids with oil. Pour in enough batter to cover two-thirds of the bottom grids. Bake according to the manufacturer's directions, but start checking for doneness after 3 minutes.

Repeat until the batter is used up; occasionally brush the grids with oil to prevent sticking.

To make the sauce: Place the strawberries, nectar, and maple syrup in a food processor. Process with on/off turns until smooth.

Drizzle the sauce over the waffles.

Serves 4

Raisin-Oat Bread

◇ *Per slice*

127 calories
0.6 g. fat
(4% of calories)
2.3 g. dietary fiber
0 mg. cholesterol
91 mg. sodium

1 large potato
2 tablespoons honey
1 cup whole wheat flour
1 cup unbleached flour
2½ teaspoons baking soda
1 teaspoon cream of tartar
¾ cup rolled oats
½ cup raisins

Peel and slice the potato. Place in a 1-quart saucepan with water to cover and cook until tender. Drain, reserving ¾ cup of the potato water. Mash the potato.

In a small bowl, combine ½ cup mashed potato, honey, and the reserved potato water. (Reserve any remaining potato for another use.)

Sift the whole wheat flour, unbleached flour, baking soda, and cream of tartar into a large bowl. Stir in the oats and raisins.

Make a well in the center of the dry ingredients and pour in the potato mixture. Stir until a stiff dough forms. Turn out onto a floured board and knead 1 minute with floured hands. Shape into a ball.

Coat an 8-inch round cake pan with nonstick spray. Add the dough and flatten slightly. With a sharp knife, make a cross slash in the top of the loaf.

Bake at 375°F for 25 to 35 minutes, or until the loaf sounds hollow when tapped. Cool completely before serving.

Makes 1 loaf; 12 slices

Prune Muffins

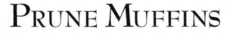

◇ *Per muffin*

127 calories
3.3 g. fat
(23% of calories)
3.9 g. dietary fiber

1 cup ready-to-eat 100% bran cereal
1½ cups buttermilk
2 egg whites
¼ cup molasses
2 tablespoons canola oil
1 teaspoon vanilla extract
1 cup whole wheat flour
½ cup oat bran
1 tablespoon baking powder
1 cup chopped prunes

1 mg. cholesterol
164 mg. sodium

*I*n a medium bowl, combine the bran cereal and buttermilk. Let stand until the cereal is soft, about 10 minutes.

Add the egg whites, molasses, oil, and vanilla. Combine well.

In a large bowl, combine the flour, oat bran, and baking powder. Stir in the prunes.

Pour the milk mixture into the flour mixture. Stir to combine, but don't overmix.

Line 12 muffin cups with cupcake papers. Spoon the batter into the cups. Bake at 400°F for about 18 minutes.

Makes 12

◇   ◇   ◇

CARROT MUFFINS

◇ *Per muffin*

165 calories
2.8 g. fat
(15% of calories)
3.6 g. dietary fiber
1 mg. cholesterol
110 mg. sodium

2 cups whole wheat flour
⅔ cup ready-to-eat bran flakes
2 teaspoons baking powder
1 teaspoon ground cinnamon

¼ teaspoon grated nutmeg
1½ cups skim milk
1½ cups shredded carrots

½ cup raisins
¼ cup egg substitute
¼ cup honey
2 tablespoons canola oil
2 tablespoons molasses

*I*n a large bowl, combine the flour, bran flakes, baking powder, cinnamon, and nutmeg.

In a medium bowl, combine the milk, carrots, raisins, egg substitute, honey, oil, and molasses.

Stir the liquid ingredients into the dry ingredients until just blended, but don't overmix.

Coat 12 muffin cups with nonstick spray. Fill about three-quarters full with the batter. Bake at 375°F for 20 to 25 minutes.

Makes 12

BANANA PANCAKES

1⅓ cups whole wheat flour
1½ teaspoons baking powder
¾ cup cooked barley
½ cup skim milk

½ cup mashed bananas
2 egg whites
2 tablespoons maple syrup
1 tablespoon canola oil

2 tablespoons all-fruit preserves
2 bananas, sliced
2 cups orange segments

*I*n a medium bowl, sift together the flour and baking powder. Stir in the barley.

In a small bowl, whisk together the milk, mashed bananas, egg whites, and maple syrup.

Pour the milk mixture into the flour. Stir to combine, but do not overmix.

Coat a well-seasoned cast-iron or nonstick frying pan with nonstick spray. Heat over medium-high heat. Add half of the oil.

Spoon in ¼ cup of the batter for each pancake. Cook until bubbles form on the top. Then flip and cook the other side for another minute. Transfer to a platter and keep warm.

Repeat with the remaining oil and batter. Transfer to the platter.

Add the preserves to the frying pan. Stir to melt. Add the bananas and oranges. Heat for 2 to 3 minutes, occasionally flipping the pieces with a spatula. Serve over the pancakes.

Serves 4

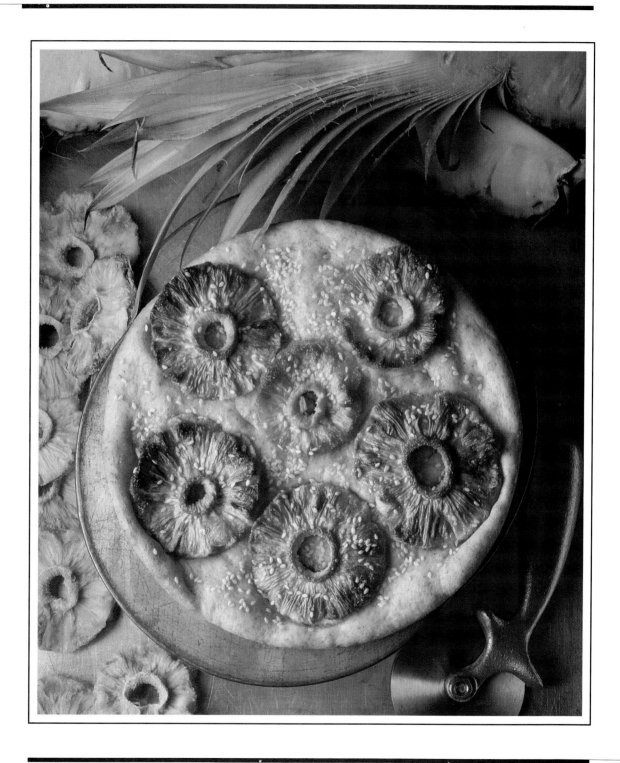

PINEAPPLE FOCCACIA (PAGE 87)

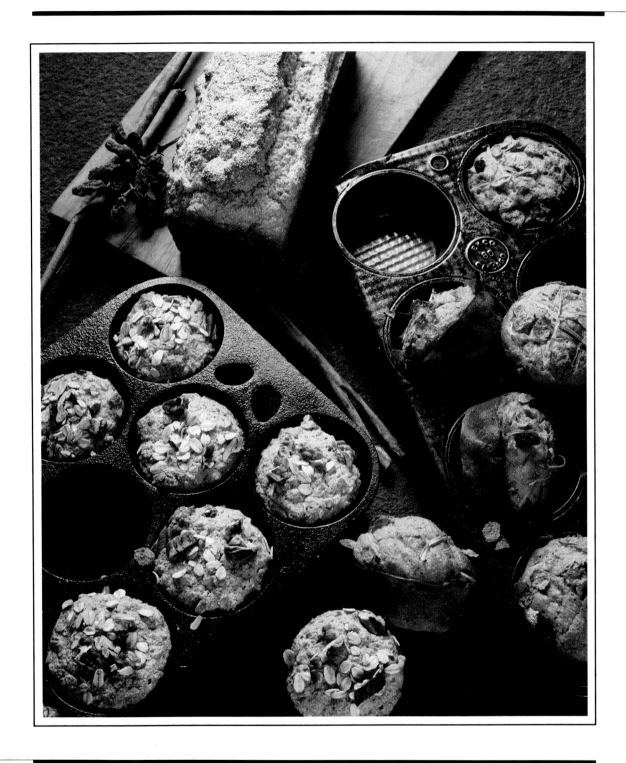

PECAN-OAT MUFFINS (PAGE 94)

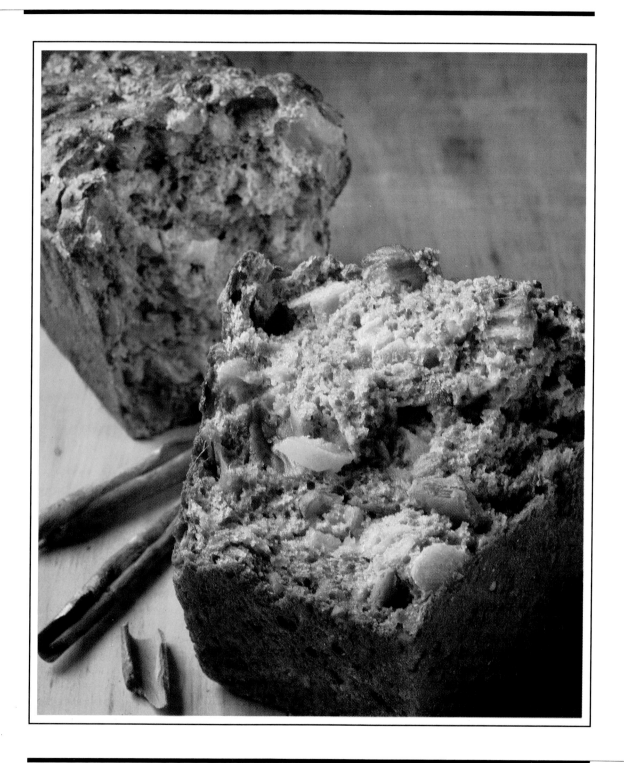

FRUIT BREAD (PAGE 92)

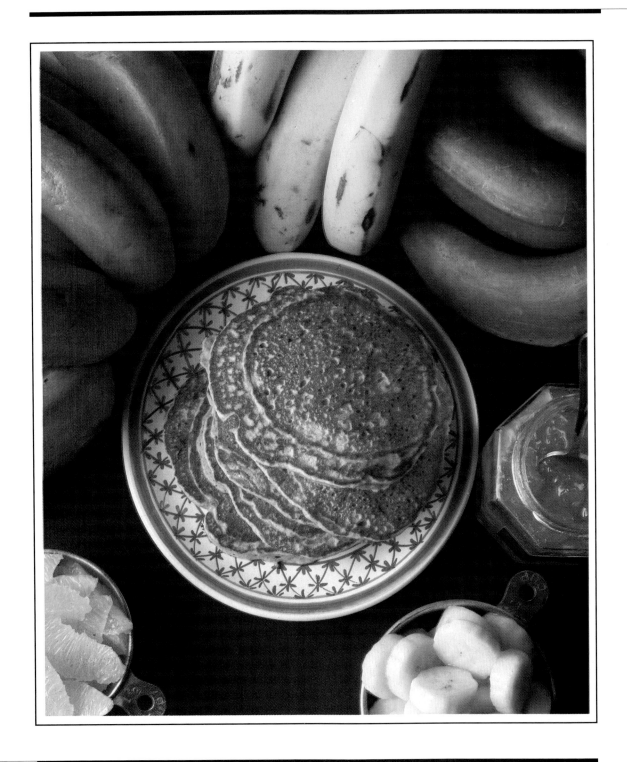

BANANA PANCAKES (PAGE 104)

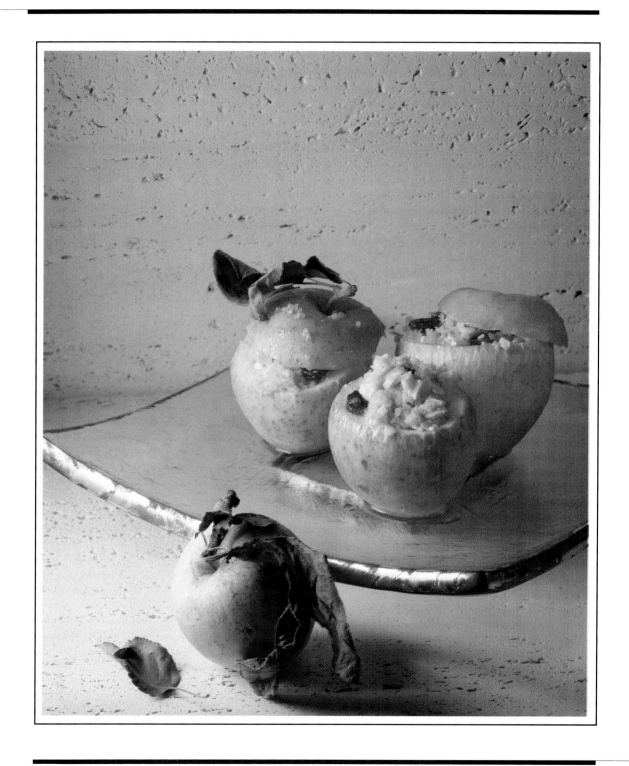

MILLET-STUFFED APPLES (PAGE 123)

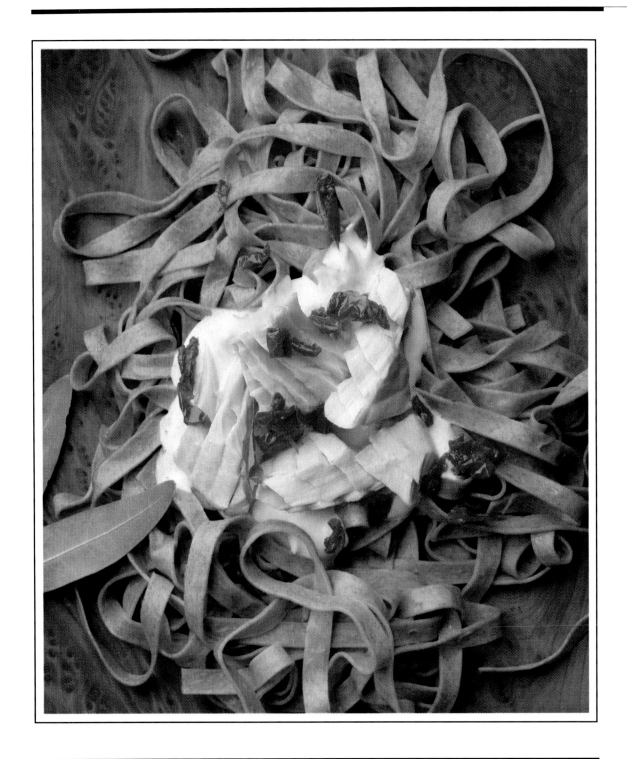

PASTA WITH SALMON AND SUN-DRIED TOMATOES (PAGE 126)

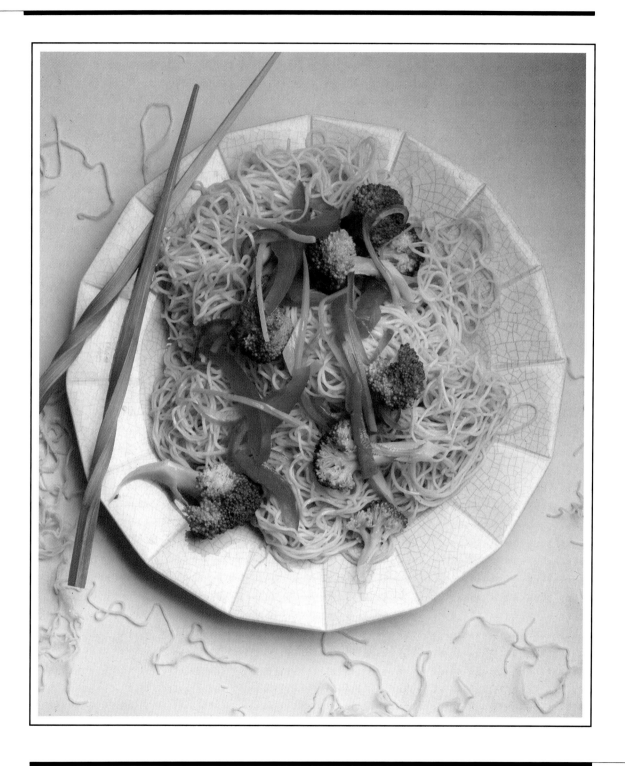

CHINESE VEGETABLE PASTA (PAGE 139)

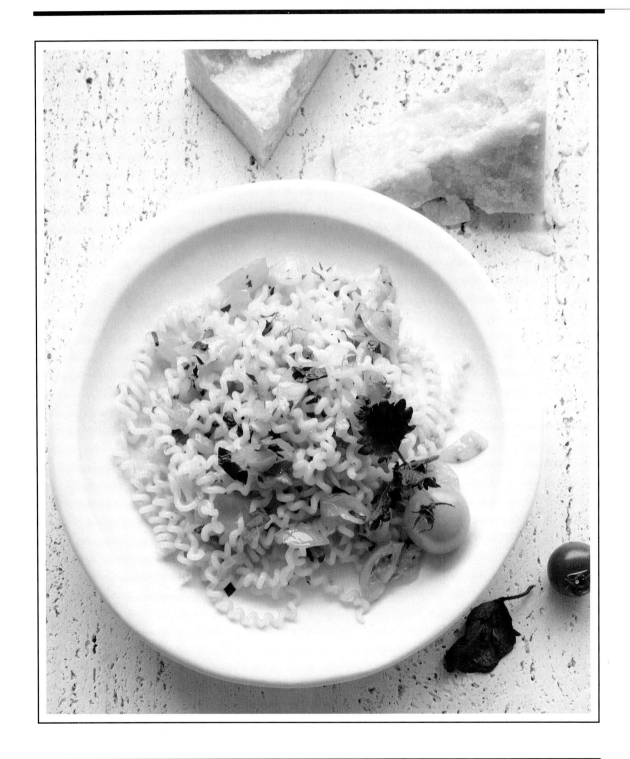

112   FUSILLI WITH FRESH TOMATO SAUCE (PAGE 136)

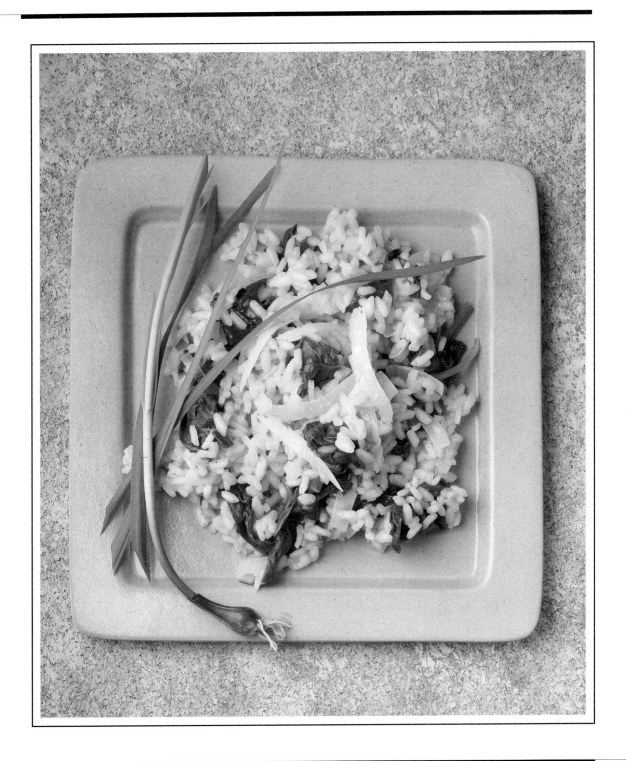

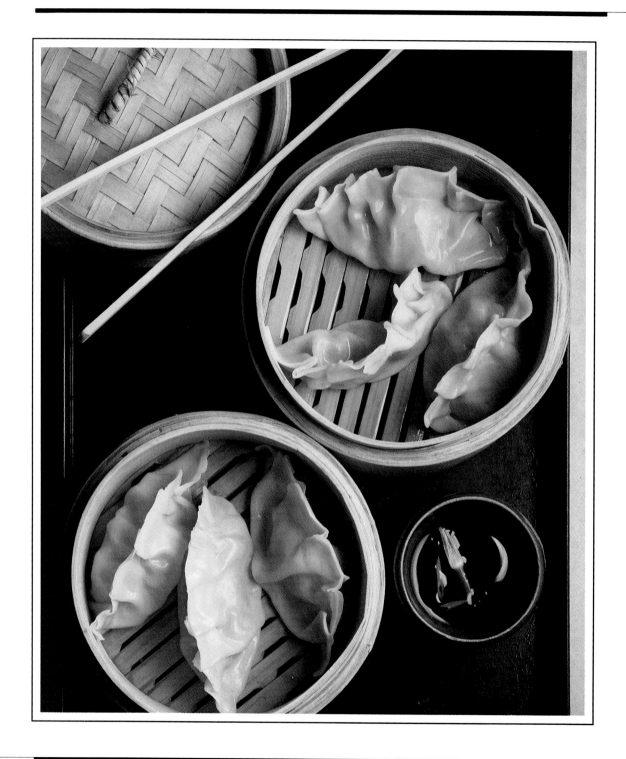

STEAMED WONTONS (PAGE 220)

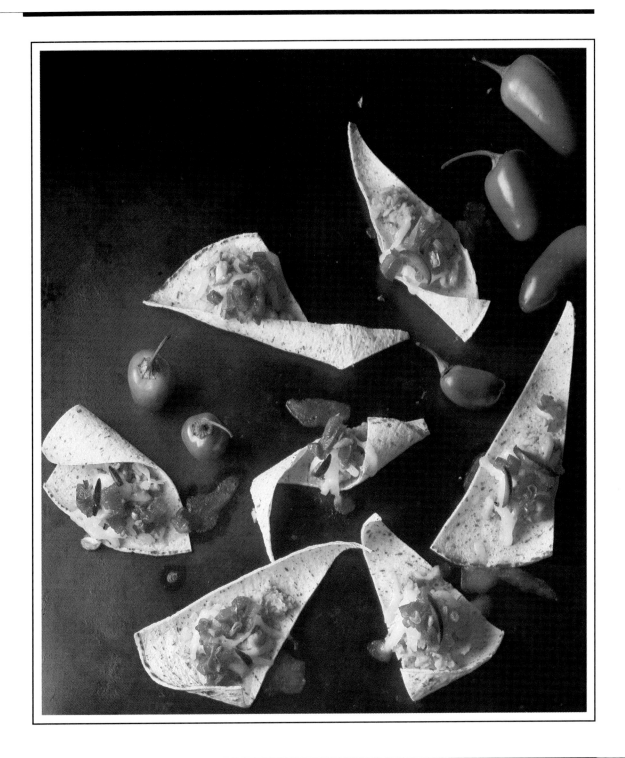

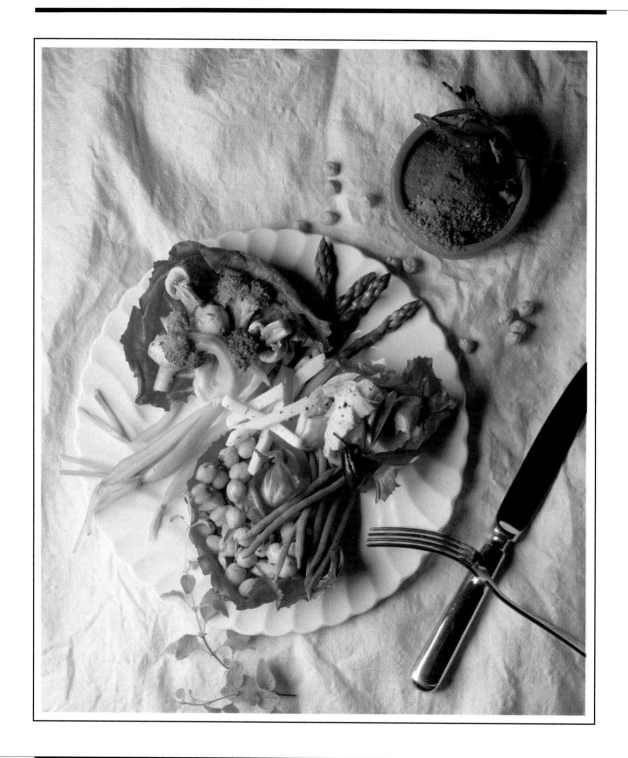

MAIN-DISH ANTIPASTO (PAGE 152)

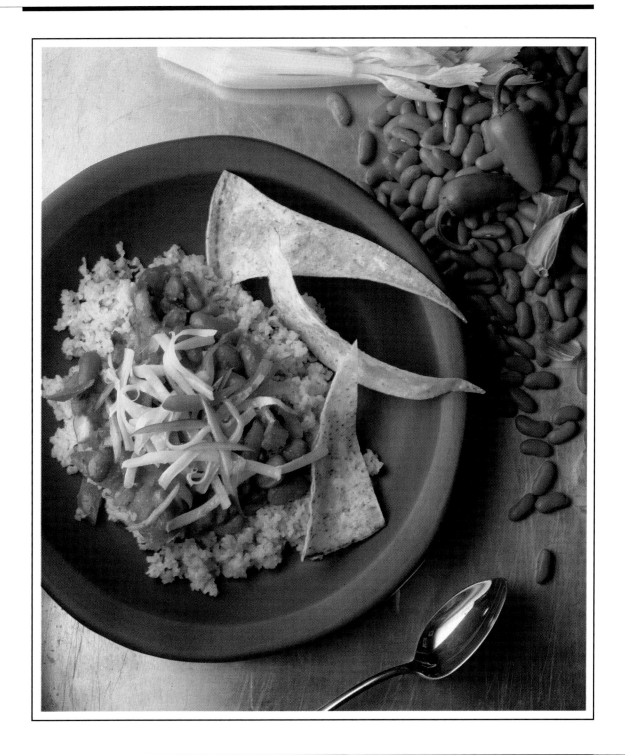

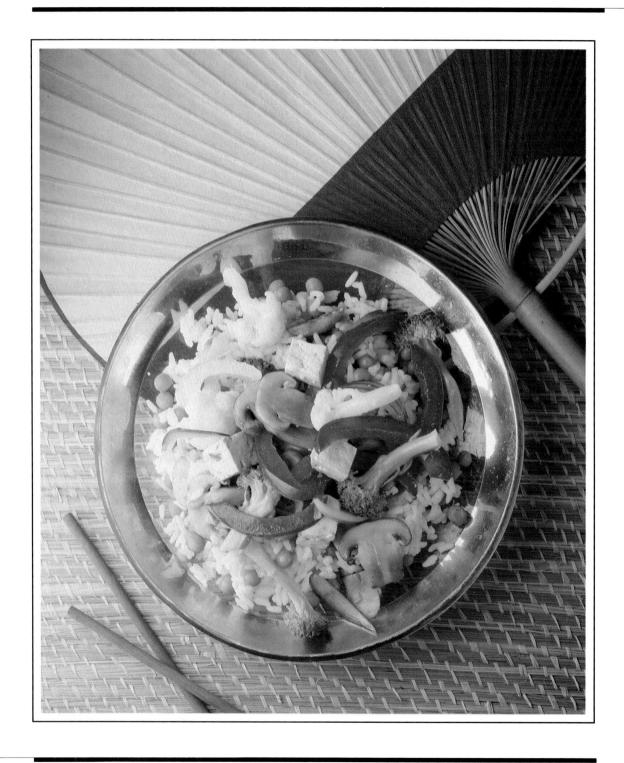

Spicy Vegetables with Tofu (page 172)

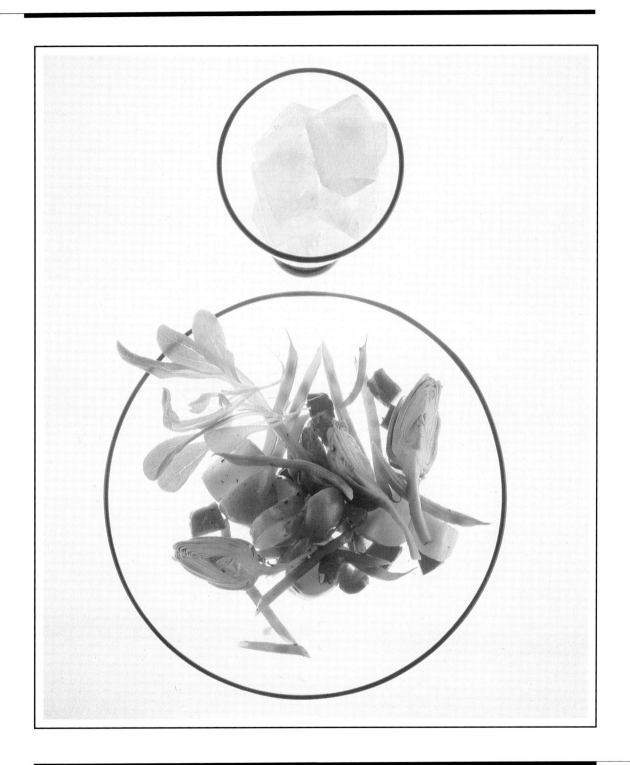

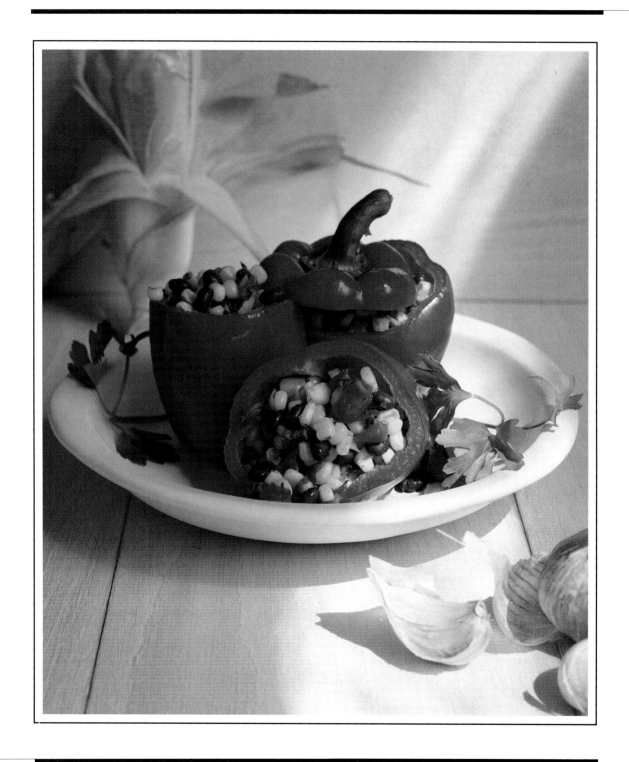

SPICY STUFFED PEPPERS (PAGE 173)

CRANBERRY BREAD

◇ *Per slice*

170 calories
0.8 g. fat
(4% of calories)
3.4 g. dietary fiber
1 mg. cholesterol
119 mg. sodium

2 cups unbleached flour
1½ cups whole wheat flour
½ cup cornmeal
1 tablespoon baking powder
½ teaspoon ground cinnamon
½ teaspoon grated nutmeg
¾ cup finely chopped cranberries
1 teaspoon anise seeds
1½ cups nonfat yogurt
¼ cup buttermilk
¼ cup egg substitute
1 tablespoon honey

Sift the unbleached flour, whole wheat flour, cornmeal, baking powder, cinnamon, and nutmeg into a large bowl. Add the cranberries and anise seeds.

In a medium bowl, combine the yogurt, buttermilk, egg substitute, and honey.

Pour the liquid ingredients into the flour bowl. Mix well, using a large rubber spatula.

Turn the dough out onto a floured counter. With floured hands, shape into a 7-inch mound, smoothing out any cracks as you go.

Coat a baking sheet with nonstick spray. Place the dough on the sheet. Use a sharp knife to slash an X in the top, about ½ inch deep (to help keep the loaf from splitting raggedly as it rises). Sprinkle the top with a bit of unbleached flour.

Bake at 450°F for about 30 minutes, or until the bottom of the bread sounds hollow when tapped. Remove from the oven and let stand about 20 minutes before slicing. Best served warm.

Makes 1 loaf; 12 slices

CHAPTER SIX ◇

The Great Grains

Grains truly are the staff of life. With lots of fiber and hunger-satisfying carbohydrates, whole grains form a very solid base for a healthy diet. Some, such as barley and oats, have been proven to help lower cholesterol. Others, such as millet and the increasingly popular quinoa, are very high in protein, making them invaluable for those who don't eat much meat. Rice is always a good low-fat choice, and buckwheat (kasha) provides a nice change of pace from the more ordinary selections.

The recipes in this chapter showcase these grains—and others—in dishes for every meal of the day. Start your morning with fruit-filled Oat-Bran Muesli or Apricot-Quinoa Cereal. Have a light lunch of Bulgur-Stuffed Yellow Peppers or Cabbage and Kasha. For a satisfying dinner, look to Skillet Barley and Beef or Spinach Risotto.

Don't forget that pasta is also a grain product. Try Pasta with Salmon and Sun-Dried Tomatoes or Buckwheat Noodles with Grilled Tuna when entertaining. (And remember that you can keep any pasta low in calories with the right sauce. Spicy Aurora Sauce, Mushroom-Cheese Sauce, and Herbed Pepper Sauce prove the point.) Fusilli with Fresh Tomato Sauce makes a nice light family dinner and is especially good with vine-ripened tomatoes.

As side dishes, Asparagus and Bulgur, Couscous with Sweet Corn, and Wild-Rice Pilaf shine. So no matter how you like your grains—sweet or savory—there's always a place for these hearty staples in the health-conscious diet.

MILLET-STUFFED APPLES

◇ *Per serving*

265 calories
3 g. fat
(10% of calories)
7.1 g. dietary fiber
5 mg. cholesterol
311 mg. sodium

½ cup millet
1 cup boiling water
4 large apples
1¼ cups low-fat cottage cheese
3 tablespoons chopped raisins
2 tablespoons shredded low-fat Muenster cheese
¼ teaspoon ground cinnamon
⅛ teaspoon grated nutmeg
½ cup water
¼ cup apple juice

*I*n a 1-quart saucepan over medium heat, toast the millet by stirring with a wooden spoon for a few minutes. Add the boiling water, cover, and simmer for 20 minutes, or until all water has been absorbed. Set aside.

Cut approximately ½ inch from the top of each apple. Remove the cores. Hollow the apples with a spoon or melon scoop, leaving sturdy shells. Finely chop 1 cup of apple pulp and set aside. (Reserve the tops and remaining pulp for another use.)

In a food processor, puree the cottage cheese until smooth. Transfer to a medium bowl. Add the chopped apples, raisins, Muenster, cinnamon, and nutmeg. Stir in the millet.

Coat an 9 × 9-inch baking dish with nonstick spray. Divide the millet mixture among the apples. Spread any remaining mixture in the bottom of the dish. Top with the apples. Add the water and apple juice to the dish. Bake at 350°F for 30 to 35 minutes, or until the apples are soft.

Serves 4

CABBAGE AND KASHA

◇ *Per serving*

188 calories
5.3 g. fat
(25% of calories)
4.9 g. dietary fiber
0 mg. cholesterol
261 mg. sodium

1 cup roasted buckwheat groats (kasha)
1 cup sliced mushrooms
3 cloves garlic, minced
5 teaspoons olive oil

2 cups defatted stock
2 teaspoons low-sodium soy sauce
1 onion, diced
4 cups shredded cabbage
1 large carrot, diced

1 sweet red pepper, diced
1½ teaspoons caraway seeds
¼ teaspoon black pepper
1 cup tomato juice

*I*n a large frying pan over medium-high heat, toast the buckwheat for 5 to 7 minutes, stirring frequently. Transfer to a bowl and set aside.

In the same frying pan, sauté the mushrooms and half of the garlic in 2 teaspoons oil for 10 minutes, or until the mushrooms are brown and no liquid is left. Add the stock, soy sauce, and buckwheat. Cover and simmer for 15 minutes, or until the buckwheat is tender. Set aside.

In another large frying pan, sauté the onions and remaining garlic in the remaining oil for 3 to 4 minutes.

Add the cabbage, carrots, peppers, caraway, and black pepper. Sauté for 5 minutes. Add the tomato juice and simmer for 15 minutes.

Arrange the buckwheat and cabbage on a large platter.

Serves 6

◇ ◇ ◇

WILD-RICE PILAF

◇ *Per serving*

173 calories
4.8 g. fat
(25% of calories)
2.3 g. dietary fiber

1 teaspoon olive oil
1 cup minced onions
1 stalk celery, minced

1 teaspoon minced garlic
¼ teaspoon red pepper
2 cups defatted chicken stock

4 ounces wild rice
1 bay leaf
2 tablespoons toasted pine nuts

*I*n a 2-quart saucepan over medium heat, heat the oil. Add the onions, celery, garlic, and pepper. Cook for 2 minutes, until lightly browned and soft.

Add the stock, wild rice, bay leaf, and pine nuts. Bring to a boil, cover, and lower the heat so the liquid simmers. Continue cooking for 55 minutes. Uncover and cook until all the liquid has been absorbed. Discard the bay leaf.

Serves 4

JAPANESE NOODLES WITH SPINACH RIBBONS

2½ ounces thin rice-stick noodles
1½ cups defatted chicken stock
1½ teaspoons dried sage
1 teaspoon low-sodium soy sauce
3 cloves garlic, minced
3 cups shredded spinach leaves
1 cup minced scallions

*I*n a large pot of boiling water, cook the noodles for 4 minutes. Drain and set aside.

In a large nonstick frying pan, combine the stock, sage, soy sauce, and garlic. Bring the mixture to a simmer.

Add the noodles. Do not stir, or the noodles will tangle; instead, gently move them around using chopsticks or tongs. When the noodles are heated, add the spinach and scallions. Simmer about 20 seconds, or until the spinach is wilted. Serve in shallow bowls.

Serves 4

Pasta with Salmon and Sun-Dried Tomatoes

1 cup water
1 tablespoon vinegar
1 bay leaf
8 ounces salmon fillet
1 cup low-fat cottage cheese

2 tablespoons skim milk
⅛ teaspoon grated nutmeg
8 ounces spinach fettuccine

⅔ cup sliced sun-dried tomatoes
1 tablespoon grated Romano cheese

*I*n a large frying pan, combine the water, vinegar, and bay leaf. Bring to a boil. Reduce the heat to low and add the salmon. Cover and cook for 4 to 6 minutes, or until opaque. Discard the bay leaf.

Remove the salmon with a slotted spoon and let cool. Break into 1-inch chunks. Set aside.

In a blender or food processor, combine the cottage cheese, milk, and nutmeg. Process until smooth.

In a large pot of boiling water, cook the fettuccine until just tender. Drain and transfer to a large serving bowl. Add the tomatoes, Romano, and half of the cottage cheese mixture. Toss to combine. Add the salmon and remaining cheese mixture. Toss gently.

Serves 4

◇

Peas and Pasta

8 ounces vermicelli
1 cup peas
1 cup sugar snap peas

¼ cup shredded low-fat Swiss cheese
¼ cup shredded part-skim mozzarella cheese

3 tablespoons minced fresh basil
¼ teaspoon grated nutmeg

*I*n a large pot of boiling water, cook the vermicelli until tender. Drain and transfer to a large bowl.

Steam the peas and snap peas for about 4 minutes, or until crisp-tender. Add to the pasta with the Swiss, mozzarella, basil, and nutmeg. Toss to combine.

Serves 4

SKILLET BARLEY AND BEEF

◇ *Per serving*

337 calories
9 g. fat
(24% of calories)
8.1 g. dietary fiber
23 mg. cholesterol
60 mg. sodium

6 ounces flank steak, trimmed of all visible fat
1 cup barley
4 cups water
1 bay leaf
1 tablespoon olive oil

1 onion, chopped
2 cloves garlic, minced
2 carrots, thinly sliced

12 mushrooms, sliced
1 ½ cups defatted beef stock
1 ½ teaspoons dried thyme

*P*artially freeze the beef (about 1 hour) to make slicing easier. Cut it lengthwise into 2-inch strips. Then slice paper thin across the grain.

In a 2-quart saucepan, combine the barley, water, and bay leaf. Bring to a boil, lower the heat, and simmer uncovered for 20 minutes.

In a large nonstick frying pan over medium heat, stir-fry the beef in the oil until cooked through, about 3 minutes. Remove from the pan and keep warm.

Add the onions and garlic to the pan. Cook until limp, about 5 minutes. Add the carrots and mushrooms; cook for 2 minutes.

Drain the barley and discard the water. Add the barley to the frying pan. Stir in the stock and thyme. Cover and simmer for 15 to 20 minutes, or until the barley is just tender.

Add the beef and warm through. Discard the bay leaf.

Serves 4

Tarragon Chicken with Linguine

◇ *Per serving*

331 calories
2.7 g. fat
(7% of calories)
3.1 g. dietary fiber
66 mg. cholesterol
113 mg. sodium

1 pound boneless, skinless chicken breasts
6 ounces linguine

1 cup defatted stock
8 mushrooms, sliced
2 carrots, julienned

1 large onion, thinly sliced
¼ cup minced fresh parsley
½ teaspoon dried tarragon

Cut the chicken into strips 3 inches long by ½ inch wide. Set aside.

Bring a large pot of water to a boil. Add the linguine and cook according to package directions until just tender. Drain and set aside.

In a large frying pan over medium heat, bring the stock to a simmer. Add the chicken and cook for 7 minutes, stirring frequently.

Add the mushrooms, carrots, onions, parsley, and tarragon. Cook until the chicken is tender, about 5 minutes.

Add the linguine to the pan. Toss to combine. Heat until the linguine is hot.

Serves 4

◇   ◇   ◇

Chili con Kasha

◇ *Per serving*

398 calories
10.1 g. fat
(23% of calories)
6.7 g. dietary fiber
36 mg. cholesterol
503 mg. sodium

8 ounces extra-lean ground beef
1 large onion, minced
1 green pepper, diced
1 clove garlic, minced

1 cup roasted buckwheat groats (kasha)
1 can (28 ounces) stewed tomatoes
1 cup tomato sauce

1 tablespoon chili powder
1 cup nonfat yogurt
½ cup chopped scallions

*I*n a large nonstick frying pan over medium-low heat, brown the beef, stirring frequently. Drain off any accumulated fat and pat the beef with a paper towel to absorb any remaining fat.

Add the onions, peppers, and garlic. Sauté until the onions are limp, about 5 minutes.

Add the buckwheat, tomatoes, tomato sauce, and chili powder. Cover and cook 20 minutes, or until the buckwheat is tender. Serve topped with the yogurt and scallions.

Serves 4

◇　　　　　　　　◇　　　　　　　　◇

PASTA PORTION GUIDE

Just how much pasta do you need to cook for tonight's spaghetti dinner or macaroni casserole? The general rule is that 2 ounces of dry pasta equals one serving. But unless you have a kitchen scale, it can be difficult to gauge just how much 2 ounces of a particular variety is without cooking the whole box, measuring the yield, and doing some long division.

So we did some of the weighing, measuring, and cooking for you to come up with portion guidelines for a handful of different pastas. This chart shows how much of each variety to measure out before cooking to serve two or four people. In most instances, 2 ounces of dry pasta turned into 1 cup cooked.

Pasta	For 2	For 4
Bow ties	2 cups	4 cups
Corn ribbons	3 cups	6 cups
Egg noodles	3 cups	6 cups
Elbow macaroni	1 cup	2 cups
Manicotti tubes	4	8
Rigatoni	2 cups	4 cups
Shells, jumbo	8	16
Shells, medium	2 cups	4 cups
Spaghetti	1-inch bunch	1½-inch bunch
Spirals	1½ cups	3 cups
Ziti	1½ cups	3 cups

CABBAGE-STUFFED SHELLS

◇ *Per serving*

276 calories
5 g. fat
(16% of calories)
3.6 g. dietary fiber
4 mg. cholesterol
336 mg. sodium

1 onion, minced
1 clove garlic, minced
1 tablespoon canola oil
2½ cups finely chopped cabbage

1 cup low-fat cottage cheese
½ teaspoon dillweed
16 jumbo shells
1 cup nonfat yogurt

1 large cucumber, shredded
1 teaspoon low-sodium soy sauce

*I*n a large nonstick frying pan, sauté the onions and garlic in the oil until soft, about 4 minutes.

Add the cabbage. Cover and cook over low heat 5 to 6 minutes, or until the cabbage is tender. Let cool for about 15 minutes.

Stir in the cottage cheese and dill.

In a large pot of boiling water, cook the shells until just tender. Drain. Stuff the shells with the cabbage mixture.

In a small bowl, combine the yogurt, cucumbers, and soy sauce. Serve the shells at room temperature with the cucumber sauce.

Serves 4

◇   ◇   ◇

BULGUR-STUFFED YELLOW PEPPERS

◇ *Per serving*

185 calories
4.3 g. fat
(21% of calories)
6 g. dietary fiber

½ cup defatted stock
½ cup bulgur
4 sweet yellow peppers
½ cup minced onion

1 tablespoon olive oil
2 cloves garlic, minced
½ teaspoon dried thyme

½ cup low-fat cottage cheese
¼ cup egg substitute
1½ cups warm tomato sauce

1 mg. cholesterol
175 mg. sodium

*I*n a 2-quart saucepan, bring the stock to a boil. Add the bulgur. Cover and remove from the heat. Set aside until the bulgur has absorbed the stock, about 20 minutes.

Slice the tops off the peppers. Remove the seeds and inner membranes. Blanch the peppers in boiling water until just tender, about 4 minutes. Set aside to cool.

In a large nonstick frying pan, combine the onions, oil, garlic, and thyme. Sauté over medium heat until the onions are tender, about 5 minutes. Add to the pan with the bulgur.

In a food processor or blender, puree the cottage cheese and egg substitute until smooth. Add to the pan with the bulgur. Combine all the ingredients well.

Divide the filling among the peppers.

Place the filled peppers in a 9 × 9-inch baking dish. Bake at 350°F for 25 minutes, or until the stuffing is firm and cooked through. Serve with the tomato sauce.

Serves 4

◇   ◇   ◇

OAT-BRAN MUESLI

◇ *Per serving*

439 calories
9.4 g. fat
(19% of calories)
13.4 g. dietary fiber
2 mg. cholesterol
100 mg. sodium

2 cups nonfat yogurt	1 banana, sliced	1 cup blackberries
2 cups rolled oats	1 orange, sectioned and chopped	
1 cup oat bran	2 kiwifruit, chopped	
¼ cup pumpkin seeds		

*I*n a large bowl, combine the yogurt, oats, and oat bran. Cover and refrigerate overnight.

Mix in the pumpkin seeds, bananas, oranges, kiwis, and blackberries.

Serves 4

SOWING THE SEEDS
OF SUCCESS

Strictly speaking, most seeds are not grains. No matter. We're including them in this chapter because they have the same earthy quality as grains. And they're an excellent, crunchy addition to most other foods. Just be aware that all seeds are not identical in nutrient profile.

Herb seeds, such as caraway, dill, anise, fennel, and coriander, pack big flavor in their small packages. Because their pronounced flavor goes a long way, you need very little in any given dish. And they add virtually no fat or calories to your diet.

Sesame and sunflower seeds, on the other hand, are much higher in fat and calories, But that's to be expected, since these seeds are often pressed to extract cooking oil. What's more, their mild flavors make it easy to consume them by the handful. Poppy seeds are similarly rich in oil. Use all these seeds as flavor accents.

Pumpkin and squash seeds fall somewhere in the middle. They're lower in fat and calories than the oil seeds but not low enough for absent-minded snacking. A few tablespoons per serving won't hurt an otherwise low-fat diet.

Here are some savory ways to use seeds.

Breads
- Combine caraway, dill, and poppy seeds. Knead into whole wheat or rye dough before letting it rise.
- Add cumin and pumpkin seeds to cornbread batter before baking.

Fish
- Toss fennel and mustard seeds into the liquid when poaching fish.
- When grilling whole fish, sprinkle the cavities with fennel and dill seeds.

Chicken
- Combine fenugreek, cumin, coriander, and fennel seeds. Pulverize and add to yogurt-based marinades.

Vegetables
- Toss cooked green beans with poppy and dill seeds.
- Sprinkle thick tomato slices with dill seeds. Broil until heated through.
- Toss cooked sweet potato chunks with toasted pumpkin seeds.

Dessert
- Add anise seeds to the liquid when poaching fruit.
- Add sesame seeds to pie crusts before baking.

APPLES AND OAT CEREAL

4 cups water
1⅓ cups oat bran
½ cup raisins
1 apple, shredded
1 tablespoon maple syrup

½ teaspoon ground caraway seeds
½ teaspoon ground cinnamon

1-2 cups skim milk

*I*n a 2-quart saucepan, bring the water and oat bran to a vigorous boil, stirring constantly. Reduce the heat to low and cook for 2 minutes, stirring frequently, until thick.

Remove from the heat and stir in the raisins, apples, maple syrup, caraway, and cinnamon. Let stand 5 minutes. Spoon into bowls and serve with the milk.

Serves 4

◇　　　　　◇　　　　　◇

SAVORY RICE PILAF

2 cups long-grain white rice
1 tablespoon olive oil

4 cups defatted stock
½ cup apple juice
1 large onion, diced

2 cloves garlic, minced
2 teaspoons lemon juice
½ teaspoon dried thyme

*I*n a 2-quart saucepan, combine the rice and oil. Stir over medium heat until the rice is golden brown, about 5 minutes.

Add the stock, apple juice, onions, garlic, lemon juice, and thyme. Bring to a boil. Reduce the heat to low, cover the pan, and simmer until all the liquid has been absorbed and the rice is tender, about 20 minutes.

Fluff with a fork before serving.

Serves 6

Couscous with Sweet Corn

1½ cups defatted chicken stock
1 cup couscous
1½ cups corn
1 cup chopped Italian tomatoes
2 cloves garlic, minced
1 teaspoon chili powder
¼ teaspoon ground cinnamon
2 tablespoons snipped chives
1 tablespoon lemon juice

*I*n a 2-quart saucepan, bring the stock to a boil. Add the couscous. Cover the pan, remove it from the heat, and let stand for about 5 minutes, or until all the liquid has been absorbed. Fluff with a fork.

In a large nonstick frying pan over medium heat, combine the corn, tomatoes, garlic, chili powder, and cinnamon. Cook until the liquid from the tomatoes evaporates, about 5 minutes. Stir in the chives and lemon juice.

Add the couscous and stir to combine.

Serves 4

◇   ◇   ◇

Barley Pilaf with Grilled Apples

PILAF
1 cup barley
2 teaspoons canola oil
1 teaspoon vanilla extract
⅛ teaspoon ground cinnamon
⅛ teaspoon grated nutmeg
⅛ teaspoon ground cardamom
1½ cups apple juice
1½ cups water

APPLES
2 baking apples
2 tablespoons apple juice
¼ teaspoon ground cinnamon

the great grains

To make the pilaf: In a 2-quart saucepan, combine the barley, oil, vanilla, cinnamon, nutmeg, and cardamom. Sauté until fragrant, about 2 minutes.

Add the apple juice and water. Bring to a boil, reduce the heat, cover, and simmer for 45 to 60 minutes, or until the barley is tender and all the liquid has been absorbed.

To make the apples: Core the apples and cut crosswise into thin rounds. Place on a baking sheet. Sprinkle with 1 tablespoon apple juice and ⅛ teaspoon cinnamon. Broil about 4 inches from the heat for about 3 minutes.

Flip the slices and sprinkle with the remaining juice and cinnamon. Grill for 2 minutes. Serve hot with the pilaf.

Serves 6

◇　　　　　　　◇　　　　　　　◇

APRICOT-QUINOA CEREAL

◇ *Per serving*

323 calories
2.7 g. fat
(8% of calories)
7.7 g. dietary fiber
1 mg. cholesterol
73 mg. sodium

1½ cups water	½ teaspoon ground cinnamon	½ cup millet
1 cup apricot nectar		¼ cup low-fat cottage cheese
1 cup chopped dried apricots	¼ teaspoon ground mace	2 tablespoons maple syrup
	½ cup quinoa	

In a 2-quart saucepan, bring the water, apricot nectar, apricots, cinnamon, and mace to a boil.

Rinse the quinoa according to the package instructions. Add the quinoa and millet to the saucepan. Reduce the heat to a simmer. Partially cover the pan and cook until the liquid is absorbed and the grains are tender, 15 to 20 minutes.

Press the cottage cheese through a sieve into a small bowl. Stir in the maple syrup. Stir the mixture into the cereal. Serve warm.

Serves 4

SPINACH RISOTTO

◇ *Per serving*

411 calories
6.7 g. fat
(15% of calories)
3.1 g. dietary fiber
2 mg. cholesterol
192 mg. sodium

5 cups defatted stock
1 tablespoon olive oil
1½ cups arborio or other short-grain rice
2 leeks, chopped
½ teaspoon curry powder
1½ cups chopped spinach
½ cup minced scallions
2 tablespoons grated Parmesan cheese

*I*n a 2-quart saucepan, bring the stock to a boil. Keep warm.

In a large nonstick frying pan over medium heat, heat the oil. Add the rice, leeks, and curry powder. Sauté for about 3 minutes.

Ladle in enough stock to just cover the rice. Simmer gently, stirring frequently, until the rice has absorbed all the stock.

Repeat, adding about 1 cup of stock at a time, until all the stock is used and the rice is tender. Do not rush the process; total cooking time should be about 25 minutes.

Stir in the spinach, scallions, and cheese. Combine well.

Serves 4

FUSILLI WITH FRESH TOMATO SAUCE

◇ *Per serving*

312 calories
8.2 g. fat
(24% of calories)
2.9 g. dietary fiber

5 tomatoes, peeled, seeded, and chopped
¼ cup chopped fresh basil
¼ cup lemon juice
2 shallots
2 tablespoons olive oil
8 ounces fusilli
1 tablespoon grated Sapsago or Parmesan cheese

0 mg. cholesterol
26 mg. sodium

*I*n a food processor or blender, process the tomatoes, basil, lemon juice, shallots, and oil until a chunky paste forms. Set aside for about 2 hours to let the flavors blend.

Cook the fusilli according to package directions until just tender. Drain well and place in a large bowl. Add the cheese and tomato sauce.

Serves 4

MICRO METHOD: Pasta Encores

Does pasta belong in the microwave? Sometimes. Although you can cook dried pasta in a microwave, it's not terribly practical. You can prepare only small amounts, and it takes just as long as—if not longer than—on the stove. What you *can* do successfully is heat or reheat dishes containing already-cooked pasta.

The power level you should use depends on whether you can stir the food or not. Something like macaroni and cheese or spaghetti and sauce can be stirred during reheating, so you can use a higher power level. When you stir the food, you move the hot food from the edges of the container to the center and thereby evenly distribute the heat.

Foods that cannot be stirred, such as lasagna, benefit from a lower power level (from 50 percent to 70 percent). That prevents the outer edges from drying out before the center is sufficiently hot.

One way to tell if your pasta dish is heated through is to carefully feel the bottom of the plate or casserole. If the container is warm, the food probably is, too. But do be careful—dishes can become quite hot in a short period of time. Always use a pot holder to lift the dish and touch the bottom gingerly.

If making casseroles, remember that food continues to cook after it's removed from the microwave. You're better off undercooking your pasta dish and letting it stand a few minutes to finish itself off. If it needs additional time in the oven after that, you can easily return it to the microwave. But it's hard to salvage a dish that's been overcooked.

Asparagus and Bulgur

◇ *Per serving*

123 calories
2.8 g. fat
(20% of calories)
5.9 g. dietary fiber
0 mg. cholesterol
7 mg. sodium

1 cup water
⅔ cup bulgur
⅓ cup thinly sliced pimientos
¼ cup vinegar
¼ cup defatted chicken stock

2 teaspoons olive oil
1 tablespoon snipped chives

1 teaspoon dried thyme
24 stalks asparagus, trimmed

*I*n a 1-quart saucepan, bring the water to a boil. Add the bulgur. Cover and let stand for 15 minutes, or until the liquid has been absorbed. Fluff with a fork.

In a large bowl, combine the pimientos, vinegar, stock, oil, chives, and thyme. Add the bulgur.

Blanch the asparagus in boiling water for 4 minutes. Slice diagonally into 2-inch sections. Add to the bulgur mixture. Combine well.

Serves 4

Buckwheat Noodles with Grilled Tuna

◇ *Per serving*

479 calories
6.2 g. fat
(12% of calories)
3.9 g. dietary fiber
51 mg. cholesterol
946 mg. sodium

2 tablespoons lemon juice
1 tablespoon olive oil
1 pound tuna steaks
1 sweet red pepper, chopped

1 tomato, peeled, seeded, and chopped
1 cup tomato juice
2 tablespoons vinegar
3 cloves garlic, minced

¼ cup minced fresh parsley
12 ounces buckwheat noodles
1 tablespoon toasted sesame seeds
3 cups shredded red lettuce

In a cup, combine the lemon juice and oil. Brush on both sides of each piece of tuna. Place in a baking dish, cover, and refrigerate for 1 hour.

Broil the tuna about 6 inches from the heat for about 5 minutes per side, or until cooked through.

In a blender, puree the peppers, tomatoes, tomato juice, vinegar, and garlic. Transfer to a small bowl and stir in the parsley.

In a large pot of boiling water, cook the noodles according to package directions until tender. Drain and place in a large bowl. Toss with the sesame seeds and half of the tomato mixture.

To serve, divide the lettuce among four dinner plates. Top with the noodles and tuna. Drizzle the fish with the remaining tomato mixture.

Serves 4

◇　　　　　　　　　◇　　　　　　　　　◇

Chinese Vegetable Pasta

1 tablespoon canola oil
1 large onion, thinly sliced
2 carrots, julienned
1 sweet red pepper, julienned

1 cup broccoli florets
1 clove garlic, thinly sliced
2 tablespoons low-sodium soy sauce
1 tablespoon vinegar

2 cups cooked vermicelli

In a large nonstick frying pan or wok, heat the oil. Add the onions and stir-fry for 2 minutes.

Add the carrots, peppers, broccoli, and garlic. Stir-fry for 2minutes.

In a small bowl, stir together the soy sauce and vinegar. Pour over the vegetables. Add the vermicelli and toss well to combine.

Serves 4

accent on Health: Sauce Sorcery

There are just two things you *never* want to do to pasta. The first is to overcook it. The second is to undermine its health potential with a fat-heavy sauce. The wrong sauce can turn a respectable 200-calorie plate of pasta into a 700-calorie diet disaster with more fat than you should eat in an entire day.

When making homemade sauce, especially cream versions, keep these tips in mind.

- Replace heavy cream with a white sauce made of low-fat or skim milk thickened with flour.
- Enrich white sauces with a little egg substitute instead of egg yolk. You'll get the same golden color and velvety texture without all the yolk's cholesterol.
- Cut back on saturated fat and cholesterol by using olive oil, canola oil, or margarine in place of butter. But remember that these fats are not lower in calories than butter, so use them judiciously.
- If making meat sauce, brown the meat first in a separate frying pan. Drain it on paper towels, and then pat it dry with more towels to draw off as much fat as possible.
- Use the lowest-fat cheeses you can find, and even then be a little stingy with them.
- Puree cooked vegetables, such as peppers, onions, or cauliflower, as low-cal thickeners for thin sauces.
- Get creamy body from well-blended low-fat or dry-curd cottage cheese. But be careful not to overheat a cottage cheese sauce, or it might curdle. Just barely warm it on the stove. Then mix with hot cooked pasta to heat it further.
- Add just enough sauce to your pasta to lightly coat it, not to smother it.

◇ ────────────────────────────

Mushroom-Cheese Sauce

1 cup low-fat cottage cheese
⅓ cup defatted chicken stock
1 teaspoon Worcestershire sauce
1 onion, minced

4 ounces mushrooms, thinly sliced
1 teaspoon olive oil
1 clove garlic, minced

the great grains

In a blender or food processor, blend the cottage cheese, stock, and Worcestershire until smooth. Set aside.

In a large nonstick frying pan over medium heat, sauté the onions and mushrooms in the oil until soft. Add the garlic and stir for 1 minute. Remove the pan from the heat. Stir in the cheese mixture. Warm over medium-low heat.

Makes 2 cups

◇*Per ½ cup:* 78 calories, 2 g. fat (23% of calories), 1 g. dietary fiber, 2 mg. cholesterol, 252 mg. sodium

◇———

Spicy Aurora Sauce

1 onion, chopped	2 cloves garlic, chopped
1 sweet red pepper, chopped	1 teaspoon dried oregano
1 tablespoon canola oil	1 cup dry-curd cottage cheese
4 cups chopped tomatoes	3 tablespoons grated Sapsago or Parmesan cheese
1 jalapeño pepper, seeded and minced	

In a large nonstick frying pan over medium heat, sauté the onions and red peppers in the oil for 5 minutes, or until soft. Add the tomatoes, jalapeño peppers, garlic, and oregano.

Cover and cook for 5 minutes, or until the tomatoes are soft and juicy. Remove the cover and cook, stirring occasionally, for 15 minutes.

Transfer to a food processor. Add the cottage cheese and puree for 2 minutes, or until the mixture is pink and no longer looks curdled.

Return the mixture to the frying pan, add the Sapsago or Parmesan, and reheat briefly. Serve immediately. (To reheat leftovers, use either very low heat or a double boiler.)

Makes 3 cups

◇*Per ½ cup:* 65 calories, 1.6 g. fat (22% of calories), 1.7 g. dietary fiber, 1 mg. cholesterol, 26 mg. sodium

(continued)

SAUCE—CONTINUED
Herbed Pepper Sauce

2 large sweet red
  peppers,
  chopped
1 large onion,
  chopped
1¼ cups defatted
  chicken stock
1 clove garlic,
  minced

1 teaspoon dried
  oregano
½ teaspoon dried
  basil
½ teaspoon dried
  savory

In a large nonstick frying pan over medium heat, cook the peppers and onions in ¼ cup stock for about 10 minutes, or until soft. Add the garlic and stir for 1 minute.

Add the remaining stock, oregano, basil, and savory. Cover and simmer for 10 minutes. Using a slotted spoon, transfer the vegetables to a blender or food processor. Add enough liquid to facilitate blending. Puree to desired consistency.

Makes 2½ cups

◇*Per ½ cup:* *31 calories, 0.6 g. fat (17% of calories), 1 g. dietary fiber, 0 mg. cholesterol, 22 mg. sodium*

CHAPTER SEVEN ◇

Beans and Legumes

W ant a first-class ticket to health? Make friends with the lowly legumes. Dried beans are such an important food that they deserve a chapter of their own. When fiber researcher James W. Anderson, M.D., conducted his landmark cholesterol studies at the University of Kentucky, his subjects consumed the amount of fiber in 1½ cups of cooked beans every day. Cholesterol levels averaging a dangerously high 294 fell by 76 points in six months.

If you're among the lucky few not worried about cholesterol, beans still have your number. They're rich in iron, B vitamins, and calcium, and they're amazingly low in fat and sodium. With no cholesterol and a hefty portion of constipation-preventing fiber, beans just seem to offer something for everybody.

There are literally dozens of types of beans to choose from, so you can have infinite variety when planning meals. The recipes in this chapter take advantage of that bounty, with dishes ranging from Chili Beans Ranchero and New Orleans Red Beans to White-Bean Gumbo and Pinto-Bean Stew. For those who love to nibble, we have a tasty selection of lean bean dips to pair with raw vegetables. Any one of them is a smart alternative to standard chips and dip when evening munchies hit.

Considering beans' sterling credentials, it's not hard to understand why they're a mainstay of almost every cuisine on the globe. And with such a wide variety of beans and bean recipes to choose from, you'll have no trouble eating the 3 to 5 cups of beans a week often recommended for optimum health.

WHITE-BEAN GUMBO

◇ *Per serving*

351 calories
2.6 g. fat
(7% of calories)
8.9 g. dietary fiber
0 mg. cholesterol
102 mg. sodium

⅓ cup whole wheat flour
3⅔ cups defatted stock
1 green pepper, finely chopped
1 stalk celery, finely chopped

1 large onion, finely chopped
2 cups chopped tomatoes
3 cloves garlic, minced
2 bay leaves

1 teaspoon dried thyme
2 cups cooked pea beans
½ teaspoon hot-pepper sauce
2 cups hot cooked rice

*P*lace the flour in a nonstick frying pan. Cook over medium-high heat, stirring constantly, until the flour is medium brown in color, about 7 minutes. Remove the pan from the heat, and pour in ⅔ cup of the stock. Whisk until smooth.

In a 3-quart saucepan, bring the remaining stock to a boil. Whisk the flour mixture into the stock. Add the peppers, celery, onions, tomatoes, garlic, bay leaves, and thyme.

Bring to a boil, then reduce the heat to a simmer. Cover the pan loosely. Simmer the gumbo, stirring occasionally, for 15 minutes. Add the drained beans and hot-pepper sauce.

Simmer until the vegetables are tender, about 15 minutes. Discard the bay leaves.

Serve over the rice.

Serves 4

◇　　　　　　　◇　　　　　　　◇

HERBED BEAN SALAD

◇ *Per serving*

266 calories
5.1 g. fat
(17% of calories)
4.5 g. dietary fiber

1 cup fresh (green) soybeans
1 cup fresh cranberry beans

2 tablespoons lime juice
2 tablespoons minced fresh mint

1 clove garlic, minced
1 large tomato, cut into 4 thick slices

0 mg. cholesterol
6 mg. sodium

Cook the soybeans and cranberry beans in boiling water to cover for 5 minutes. Drain and place in a large bowl.

Add the lime juice, mint, and garlic. Chill.

Divide the tomatoes among individual salad plates. Top with the beans.

Serves 4

◇ ◇ ◇

Mexican Bean Pie

◇ *Per serving*

286 calories
6.8 g. fat
(21% of calories)
9.5 g. dietary fiber
4 mg. cholesterol
170 mg. sodium

4 corn tortillas
½ cup sliced scallions
2 green peppers, diced
2 cloves garlic, minced
1 tablespoon olive oil

2 cups cooked pinto beans, mashed
2 tomatoes, chopped
2 teaspoons chili powder
1 teaspoon ground coriander

¾ cup egg substitute
¼ cup shredded low-fat Monterey Jack cheese

Heat the tortillas at 350°F for 5 to 8 minutes, or until crispy. Break into pieces, then pulverize in a blender.

Coat four 5-inch pie pans with nonstick spray. Coat with the tortilla crumbs. Reserve any extra.

In a large nonstick frying pan, sauté the scallions, peppers, and garlic in the oil until tender, about 5 minutes.

Add the beans, tomatoes, chili powder, and coriander. Sauté for 5 minutes.

Remove from the heat and stir in the egg substitute. Divide among the prepared pans. Sprinkle with reserved crumbs.

Bake at 375°F for 20 minutes.

Top with the cheese.

Serves 4

BLACK BEANS AND RICE

◇ *Per serving*

335 calories
4.5 g. fat
(12% of calories)
6.1 g. dietary fiber
1 mg. cholesterol
58 mg. sodium

1 tablespoon olive oil
2 sweet red peppers, finely chopped
1 large onion, finely chopped
1 stalk celery, finely chopped

2 cloves garlic, minced
¼ teaspoon dried thyme
2 cups cooked black beans
2 tablespoons apple-cider vinegar

2 cups hot cooked rice
1 cup nonfat yogurt

*H*eat the oil in a large nonstick frying pan. Add the peppers, onions, celery, garlic, and thyme. Sauté over medium heat until the vegetables are fragrant and tender, about 10 minutes.

Add the beans and vinegar. Cook until the beans are hot, about 3 minutes.

To serve, divide the rice among shallow bowls. Top with the beans and yogurt.

Serves 4

MICRO METHOD: No More All-Nighters

Here's an easy way to soak beans that doesn't take all night. Rinse 1 pound of dried beans. Place in a 5-quart micro-safe casserole with 6 or 7 cups of cold water. Microwave on full power for 8 to 10 minutes, or until the water boils. Boil for 2 minutes. Let the beans stand for 1 hour before proceeding with your recipe.

Because dried beans must slowly absorb water to become tender, they won't cook any more quickly in the microwave than atop the stove.

One thing to keep in mind when buying dried beans and other legumes, such as lentils: Look for bright colors and uniform size. Dullness indicates long storage, which will markedly prolong cooking time no matter what method you use. And beans of different sizes won't cook at the same speed, leaving you with some that are either overcooked or still tough.

New Orleans Red Beans

1 pound dried red beans, soaked overnight
6 cups water
1 large onion, chopped
1 green pepper, chopped
¼ cup minced fresh parsley
4 cloves garlic, minced
1 small hot chili pepper, seeded and minced
½ teaspoon crushed red-pepper flakes
⅛ teaspoon ground red pepper
2 bay leaves
1 teaspoon dried thyme
1 teaspoon dried basil
3 cups hot cooked rice

*D*rain the beans. In a 4-quart pot, combine the beans, water, onions, green peppers, parsley, garlic, chili peppers, pepper flakes, ground pepper, bay leaves, thyme, and basil.

Cover and bring to boil over medium heat. Reduce the heat to low and cook for 3 to 4 hours, or until the beans are tender. Stir occasionally as the beans cook. Most of the water will be absorbed; if necessary, add a little more water during cooking to keep the mixture from sticking. Discard the bay leaves.

Serve over the rice.

Serves 6

Chick-Pea Chili

◇ *Per serving*

448 calories
6.9 g. fat
(14% of calories)
7.7 g. dietary fiber
1 mg. cholesterol
110 mg. sodium

1 large onion, minced
2 cloves garlic, minced
1 tablespoon olive oil
2 cups cooked chick-peas
1½ cups tomato sauce
1 tablespoon chili powder
1 teaspoon ground cumin
½ teaspoon dried oregano
⅛ teaspoon red pepper
2 cups hot cooked rice
1 cup nonfat yogurt
1 cup diced green peppers
1 cup diced tomatoes
1 cup shredded lettuce

*I*n a 2-quart saucepan over medium heat, cook the onions and garlic in the oil until translucent. Stir in the chick-peas, tomato sauce, chili powder, cumin, oregano, and red pepper. Simmer, uncovered, about 30 minutes.

Serve over the rice topped with the yogurt, peppers, tomatoes, and lettuce.

Serves 4

Great Northern Soup

◇ *Per serving*

229 calories
5 g. fat
(20% of calories)
8.1 g. dietary fiber
0 mg. cholesterol
115 mg. sodium

1 cup dried Great Northern beans, soaked overnight
1 large onion, chopped
1 green pepper, chopped
1 stalk celery, chopped
1 carrot, chopped
2 cloves garlic, chopped
1 tablespoon canola oil
2 cups defatted chicken stock
½ cup orange juice
1 teaspoon low-sodium soy sauce
¼ teaspoon ground cumin
2 tablespoons lemon juice
¼ cup snipped chives

*D*rain the beans. Place in a 4-quart saucepan with water to cover. Cover the pan and simmer until the beans are almost tender, about 1½ hours. Drain and transfer to a bowl.

In the same pan, sauté the onions, peppers, celery, carrots, and garlic in the oil until tender.

Add the beans, stock, orange juice, soy sauce, and cumin. Cover and simmer until the beans are tender, about 45 to 60 minutes. Remove from the heat and cool slightly.

Working in batches, puree the soup in a blender or food processor. Return it to the pan. Add the lemon juice and heat briefly. Serve sprinkled with the chives.

Serves 4

◇　　　　　　　　　　◇　　　　　　　　　　◇

Mushroom and Lentil Soup

◇ *Per serving*

130 calories
3.6 g. fat
(25% of calories)
3.1 g. dietary fiber
0 mg. cholesterol
75 mg. sodium

1 large onion, chopped
1 tablespoon olive oil
5 cups defatted stock

8 ounces mushrooms, sliced
1 carrot, diced
½ cup dried lentils

1 teaspoon dried rosemary
1 bay leaf

*I*n a 3-quart saucepan over medium heat, sauté the onions in the oil until lightly browned, about 12 to 15 minutes.

Add the stock, mushrooms, carrots, lentils, rosemary, and bay leaf. Bring to a boil. Reduce the heat, cover loosely, and let simmer until the lentils are tender, about 30 minutes.

Discard the bay leaf.

Serves 6

Vegetable Chili

◇ *Per serving*

367 calories
8.4 g. fat
(20% of calories)
10.8 g. dietary fiber
0 mg. cholesterol
337 mg. sodium

2 tablespoons olive oil
2 cups finely chopped onions
2 cups diced celery
2 cups diced carrots
1 sweet red pepper, diced
4 cloves garlic, minced

2 tablespoons whole wheat flour
1 tablespoon chili powder
4 cups crushed tomatoes
1½ cups defatted stock
1 cup dried adzuki beans, soaked overnight

*I*n a 4-quart pot, heat the oil. Add the onions, celery, carrots, peppers, and garlic. Sauté for 5 to 10 minutes, or until tender. Stir in the flour and chili powder.

Add the tomatoes, stock, and drained beans.

Cover and simmer for 30 minutes. Remove the lid and simmer 30 minutes, or until the vegetables and beans are tender and the liquid has thickened.

Serves 4

Caspian Split Peas

◇ *Per serving*

159 calories
1.7 g. fat
(10% of calories)
5.3 g. dietary fiber

4 cups defatted stock
2 large tomatoes, diced

2 carrots, thinly sliced
1 cup shredded cabbage
½ cup green split peas

½ cup barley
2 cloves garlic, minced
¼ cup minced fresh parsley

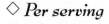

*I*n a 4-quart pot, combine the stock, tomatoes, carrots, cabbage, split peas, barley, and garlic.

Bring to a boil, reduce the heat to medium-low, cover, and simmer for about 1¼ hours, or until the barley is tender.

Stir in the parsley.

Serves 6

◇   ◇   ◇

PINTO-BEAN STEW

◇ *Per serving*

300 calories
5.1 g. fat
(15% of calories)
13.2 g. dietary fiber
0 mg. cholesterol
98 mg. sodium

1 large onion, thinly sliced
1 clove garlic, minced
1 tablespoon dried oregano
1 tablespoon chili powder
2 teaspoons canola oil

2 cups chopped tomatoes
3 cups defatted stock
1 cup dried pinto beans, soaked overnight

1 green pepper, diced
1½ cups cubed pumpkin
1 cup corn

*I*n a large nonstick frying pan, sauté the onions, garlic, oregano, and chili powder in the oil for 3 to 4 minutes. Add the tomatoes and cook for 5 minutes.

Transfer to a 3-quart casserole dish. Add the stock and drained beans. Cover and bake at 375°F for 1½ hours.

Add the peppers, pumpkin, and corn. Bake for 1 hour, or until the beans and vegetables are tender.

Lightly mash about half of the beans before serving to help thicken the stew.

Serves 4

MAIN-DISH ANTIPASTO

◇ *Per serving*

459 calories
10.5 g. fat
(21% of calories)
12.9 g. dietary fiber
17 mg. cholesterol
521 mg. sodium

MARINADE
2 tablespoons olive oil
2 tablespoons rice-wine vinegar
2 tablespoons herb vinegar
1 tablespoon minced fresh parsley
½ teaspoon dry mustard
½ teaspoon dried oregano
¼ teaspoon paprika
⅛ teaspoon black pepper

ANTIPASTO
¾ cup cooked chick-peas or kidney beans
1 slice onion
1 clove garlic, halved
1 sweet red pepper
24 green beans, trimmed
2 large carrots, julienned
12 mushrooms

2 large stalks broccoli
12 asparagus spears
4 cubes part-skim mozzarella cheese
4 black olives
1 can (7½ ounces) water-packed tuna
8 slices Italian bread

*T*o make the marinade: In a small bowl, whisk together the oil, rice-wine vinegar, herb vinegar, parsley, mustard, oregano, paprika, and pepper.

To make the antipasto: Place the chick-peas or kidney beans in a small bowl. Add 3 to 4 tablespoons of marinade and toss to coat. Top with the onion and garlic. Cover and refrigerate until needed.

Broil the pepper 3 to 4 inches from the heat until charred on all sides. Wrap the pepper in a damp dish towel and set aside for 5 minutes. Peel off the blackened skin and discard the seeds. Cut the flesh into thin strips. Set aside.

Arrange the green beans in half of a large steaming basket. Arrange the carrots in the other half. Cover and steam over 1 inch of boiling water for 4 to 5 minutes, or until crisp-tender. Rinse under cold water to stop the cooking, pat dry, and set aside.

Steam the mushrooms for 8 to 10 minutes, or until cooked through. Pat dry and set aside.

Peel the tough skin away from the broccoli stems. Cut the broccoli into florets, leaving 2 inches of stem intact. Steam for 2 to 3 minutes, or until crisp-tender. Rinse under cold water, pat dry, and set aside.

Trim the woody ends from the asparagus. With a vegetable peeler, remove the scales from the spears. Steam the asparagus for 3 to 5 minutes, or until crisp-tender. Run under cold water, pat dry, and set aside.

When ready to serve, remove and discard the onion and garlic from the chick-peas or kidney beans. Toss the chick-peas or kidney beans with their dressing, then drain and save the marinade.

For a decorative presentation, arrange the vegetables on a large serving platter in this order: broccoli, mushrooms, carrots, green beans, peppers, asparagus. Spoon the marinade from the chick-peas or kidney beans over the vegetables. Whisk the remaining marinade and drizzle over the platter. Add the cheese, olives, and chick-peas or kidney beans.

Open the can of tuna and press out excess liquid with the can lid. Invert the can and turn the tuna out onto the platter in one piece.

Serve the antipasto at room temperature with the bread.

Serves 4

Nachos

◇ *Per serving*

351 calories
6.8 g. fat
(17% of calories)
9.5 g. dietary fiber
5 mg. cholesterol
409 mg. sodium

12 corn tortillas
1½ cups cooked pinto beans

1 cup salsa
1 cup minced sweet red peppers

½ cup shredded low-fat Monterey Jack cheese

Cut the tortillas into quarters. Place the pieces on a baking sheet and bake at 400° F until crisp but not brown, about 5 minutes. Let cool for a few minutes.

Coarsely mash the beans. Spread the beans on the tortillas and return the wedges to the baking sheet. Dot with the salsa. Sprinkle with the peppers and cheese.

Bake until the cheese has melted, about 3 minutes. Serve warm.

Serves 4

Variation:
■ Before the second baking, sprinkle the tortillas with minced jalapeño peppers, minced sweet red peppers, or minced black olives.

Good-Luck Peas

◇ *Per serving*

162 calories
4 g. fat
(22% of calories)
7.6 g. dietary fiber
0 mg. cholesterol
35 mg. sodium

2 cups cooked black-eyed peas
2 cups shredded carrots
1 cup shredded kale
1 cup minced leeks

2 tablespoons lemon juice
2 tablespoons red-wine vinegar
1 tablespoon olive oil
1 teaspoon dried basil

½ teaspoon dried sage
¼ teaspoon dry mustard

In a large bowl, combine the peas, carrots, kale, and leeks.

In a small bowl, whisk together the lemon juice, vinegar, oil, basil, sage, and mustard. Pour over the peas and toss to combine.

Serves 4

CHILI BEANS RANCHERO

◇ *Per serving*

323 calories
2.7 g. fat
(8% of calories)
16.4 g. dietary fiber
3 mg. cholesterol
76 mg. sodium

1 pound dried kidney beans, soaked overnight
6 cups water
2 cups tomato sauce
4 scallions, thinly sliced
2 stalks celery, finely chopped
2 carrots, finely chopped
2 onions, diced
1 tomato, diced
1 sweet red pepper, diced
2 small chili peppers, seeded and minced
¼ cup minced fresh parsley
5 cloves garlic, minced
1 tablespoon chili powder
2 teaspoons paprika
1½ teaspoons dried oregano
1 teaspoon dried marjoram
1 teaspoon ground cumin
¼ teaspoon ground red pepper
2 bay leaves
4–5 cups hot cooked bulgur
½ cup shredded low-fat Cheddar cheese

*D*rain the beans and place in 4-quart pot. Add the water. Cover and bring to a simmer over medium heat. Turn the heat to low and cook for 1 hour.

Add the tomato sauce, scallions, celery, carrots, onions, tomatoes, red peppers, chili peppers, parsley, garlic, chili powder, paprika, oregano, marjoram, cumin, ground red pepper, and bay leaves. Cover and simmer for 1 hour. Discard the bay leaves.

Serve over the bulgur. Sprinkle with the cheese.

Serves 8

Black-Eyed Peas with Spinach

2 tablespoons vinegar
2 teaspoons olive oil
1 teaspoon Dijon mustard
1 clove garlic, minced
¼ teaspoon dried oregano

¼ teaspoon dried basil
⅛ teaspoon grated nutmeg
2 cups shredded spinach

1½ cups cooked black-eyed peas
2 plum tomatoes, chopped
1 small onion, thinly sliced

In a small bowl, whisk together the vinegar, oil, and mustard. Stir in the garlic, oregano, basil, and nutmeg.

In a large bowl, combine the spinach, peas, tomatoes, and onions. Pour on the dressing and toss well to combine.

Serves 4

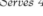

Navy-Bean Soup

¾ cup dried navy beans, soaked overnight
6 cups defatted beef stock
1 cup chopped tomatoes
3 parsnips, diced

2 onions, coarsely chopped
2 yellow frying peppers, diced
5 cloves garlic, minced

1 teaspoon dried thyme
½ teaspoon caraway seeds
2 tablespoons red-wine vinegar

beans and legumes

*D*rain the beans. Place in a 4-quart pot with the stock. Simmer for 25 minutes.

Add the tomatoes, parsnips, onions, peppers, garlic, thyme, and caraway.

Cover and simmer until the beans are tender, about 20 minutes. Crush some of the beans with a potato masher to thicken the soup.

Stir in the vinegar.

Serves 6

◇   ◇   ◇

DIP INTO SOMETHING HEALTHY

Beans make a great alternative to cheese spreads and sour cream dips for those on a heart-healthy diet. In addition to being low in fat, their high fiber content will help make a little go a long way when it comes to appeasing your appetite. That means bean dips are perfect for the weight watcher, too!

The basic directions are the same for all the dips that follow.

■ If cooking your own beans, make sure they're very soft so you can mash them easily. Drain the beans, but save at least ½ cup of the liquid.

■ If using canned beans, drain them and reserve the liquid. Place the beans themselves in a strainer and rinse under cold water to remove excess sodium.

■ Transfer the beans to a blender or food processor. Process them until smooth, adding only enough liquid to facilitate blending.

■ Stir in the listed condiments and spices. (If you want to try combinations of your own, use approximately 2 teaspoons of seasoning plus 2 tablespoons of condiments or chopped vegetables for each cup of beans.)

■ Serve your spreads on toasted pita chips, whole-grain crackers, corn tortillas (cut into sixths and toasted), or crudités (bite-size broccoli, cauliflower, carrots, mushrooms, celery, or other cut fresh vegetables).

(continued)

Chili Bean Dip

1 cup cooked
  pink beans
1 teaspoon chili
  powder
1 teaspoon onion
  powder

1 teaspoon
  chopped green
  chili peppers
¼ teaspoon red
  pepper

Makes about 1 cup

◇*Per ¼ cup:* *63 calories, 0.4 g. fat (6% of calories),
3.2 g. dietary fiber, 0 mg. cholesterol, 7 mg. sodium*

◇────────────────────────

Creole Bean Dip

1 cup cooked red
  beans
2 tablespoons
  finely chopped
  green peppers

2 tablespoons
  minced tomatoes
5 drops hot-
  pepper sauce

Makes about 1 cup

◇*Per ¼ cup:* *58 calories, 0.3 g. fat (5% of calories),
4.1 g. dietary fiber, 0 mg. cholesterol, 16 mg. sodium*

◇────────────────────────

Coriander-Bean Dip

1 cup cooked red
  beans
1 teaspoon
  ground
  coriander

1 teaspoon
  ground cumin

Makes about 1 cup

◇*Per ¼ cup:* *58 calories, 0.2 g. fat (3% of calories),
3.5 g. dietary fiber, 0 mg. cholesterol, 3 mg. sodium*

beans and legumes

Red-Pepper Bean Spread

1 cup cooked
  Great Northern
  beans
3 tablespoons
  finely chopped
  sweet red
  peppers

1 tablespoon
  finely chopped
  scallions

Makes about 1 cup

◇*Per ¼ cup: 54 calories, 0.3 g. fat (5% of calories),
2.5 g. dietary fiber, 0 mg. cholesterol, 3 mg. sodium*

Beans Florentine

1 cup Great
  Northern beans
2 tablespoons
  chopped
  cooked spinach
  (squeezed dry)

½ teaspoon dried
  thyme
½ teaspoon onion
  powder

Makes about 1 cup

◇*Per ¼ cup: 54 calories, 0.3 g. fat (5% of calories),
2.5 g. dietary fiber, 0 mg. cholesterol, 3 mg. sodium*

Curried Pea Spread

1 cup cooked
  peas

½–1 teaspoon
  curry powder

Makes about 1 cup

◇*Per ¼ cup: 30 calories, 0.2 g. fat (6% of calories),
1.8 g. dietary fiber, 0 mg. cholesterol, 93 mg. sodium*

CUBAN BEAN STEW

◇ *Per serving*

147 calories
1.9 g. fat
(12% of calories)
4.3 g. dietary fiber
0 mg. cholesterol
245 mg. sodium

½ cup dried black beans, soaked overnight
4 cups defatted chicken stock
1 large onion, chopped
1 stalk celery, thinly sliced
2 hot chili peppers, seeded and minced
¼ cup minced fresh parsley
1 tablespoon peeled minced gingerroot
1 tablespoon low-sodium soy sauce
4 cloves garlic, minced
1 teaspoon dried thyme
1 bay leaf

*D*rain the beans. Place in a 3-quart casserole dish. Add the stock, onions, celery, peppers, parsley, ginger, soy sauce, garlic, thyme, and bay leaf.

Bring to a simmer on top of the stove.

Transfer to the oven and bake at 375°F for 2 hours, or until the beans are tender. Discard the bay leaf.

Serves 4

◇ ◇ ◇

GRILLED TILEFISH WITH BEAN SALSA

◇ *Per serving*

289 calories
6.9 g. fat
(21% of calories)
5.2 g. dietary fiber
0 mg. cholesterol
74 mg. sodium

2 cups cooked black beans
2 large tomatoes, diced
1 large onion, diced
½ cup minced fresh coriander
3 tablespoons vinegar
1 tablespoon minced chili peppers
¼ cup defatted stock
2 tablespoons lime juice
1 tablespoon olive oil
1 teaspoon black pepper
2 cloves garlic, minced
1 pound tilefish fillets

*I*n a 2-quart saucepan, combine the beans, tomatoes, onions, coriander, vinegar, and peppers. Cover and let stand about 30 minutes.

In a small bowl, whisk together the stock, lime juice, oil, black pepper, and garlic.

Place the fish in a shallow baking dish. Pour the oil mixture over it. Cover, refrigerate, and marinate for 30 minutes.

Coat a broiler rack with nonstick spray. Transfer the fish directly to the rack. Broil about 4 inches from the heat for 5 to 7 minutes per side, or until cooked through. Transfer to serving plates.

While the fish is cooking, heat the bean mixture for a few minutes, until just warm. Serve with the fish.

Serves 4

◇　　　　　　　◇　　　　　　　◇

Red Beans in Edible Cups

2 cups cooked kidney beans
2 cups cooked yellow beans, cut into 1-inch pieces
2 large tomatoes, diced

2 shallots, minced
1 tablespoon snipped chives
1 teaspoon dried basil
2 tablespoons vinegar

2 tablespoons olive oil
12 small purple cabbage leaves

*I*n a large bowl, combine the drained kidney beans, yellow beans, tomatoes, shallots, chives, and basil.

In a cup, whisk together the vinegar and oil. Pour over the bean mixture. Toss well to combine.

To serve, place the cabbage leaves on individual plates. Divide the beans among them.

Serves 4

CHAPTER EIGHT ◇

Vegetarian Main Meals

ant to bask in good health? Become a vegetarian. Long-term studies of Seventh-Day Adventists, who advocate vegetarianism, show that they have half the death rate from heart disease as the national average. The fact that Adventists also shun cigarettes and alcohol no doubt plays a part in their better-than-average heart disease rate. But their no-meat—meaning low-fat—lifestyle definitely works greatly in their favor, according to researchers.

This doesn't mean that *you* have to shun meat forever to garner similar health benefits. But you could eat meat less often. After all, any healthy diet should contain a fair share of vegetarian dishes. Why? Because fruits and vegetables, especially the rich green and yellow varieties, are storehouses of valuable nutrients that fight heart disease and cancer. They also provide the beneficial fiber so important to digestive health.

Dishes in this chapter emphasize ingredients such as grains, tofu, legumes, and egg substitute, which provide the protein often lacking in a meatless regime. What's more, these recipes are filling and hearty. A number of recipes also feature fiber-filled corn, which is a staple in cuisines that rely less heavily on meat than the standard American diet. Try Mexican Corn Casserole, Corn Enchiladas, or one of the many variations of polenta, a versatile Italian staple.

What more could you ask from a cuisine that's so naturally nutritious? Well, how about low fat and low calories? After all, when was the last time you saw a fat vegetarian!

ACORN SQUASH STUFFED WITH CORNBREAD

◇ *Per serving*

361 calories
9.9 g. fat
(25% of calories)
9.6 g. dietary fiber
<1 mg. cholesterol
177 mg. sodium

CORNBREAD
- ¾ cup yellow cornmeal
- ½ cup whole wheat flour
- 1½ teaspoons baking powder
- ½ cup skim milk
- ¼ cup egg substitute
- 1 tablespoon honey
- ¼ cup chopped pecans

SQUASH
- 2 large acorn squash
- 1 tablespoon olive oil
- 1 teaspoon dried basil
- 1 teaspoon grated nutmeg
- ½ cup apple juice

*T*o make the cornbread: In a large bowl, mix the cornmeal, flour, and baking powder. In a small bowl, mix the milk, egg substitute, and honey. Pour the liquid ingredients into the flour mixture and stir lightly. Fold in the pecans until all the flour is moistened. Do not overmix.

Coat a 9 × 5-inch loaf pan with nonstick spray. Add the batter. Bake at 350°F for 15 minutes. Allow the bread to cool.

To make the squash: Cut the squash in half lengthwise. Scoop out and discard the seeds. Coat a 9 × 13-inch baking dish with nonstick spray. Add the squash, cut-side down. Add a small amount of water to the pan so the squash won't stick during baking.

Bake at 350°F for 45 to 60 minutes, or until just tender. Do not overbake, or the squash will collapse.

Allow the squash to cool slightly. Scoop out the flesh, leaving a ½-inch shell. Transfer the pulp to a large bowl.

Crumble the cornbread and add to the bowl. Add the oil, basil, and nutmeg. Toss lightly to mix. Add the apple juice and mash lightly with a potato masher. Do not overmix; stuffing should be slightly lumpy. If necessary, add a bit more juice to make a moist mixture.

Mound the stuffing in the squash shells. Bake at 350°F for 15 minutes, or until heated through.

Serves 4

SPINACH AND FETA PIE

◇ *Per serving*

123 calories
2.8 g. fat
(20% of calories)
3.5 g. dietary fiber
4 mg. cholesterol
292 mg. sodium

1 pound spinach
1 cup egg substitute
½ cup nonfat yogurt
2 tablespoons crumbled feta cheese

2 cloves garlic, minced
1 teaspoon dried oregano
½ teaspoon ground cinnamon

⅓ cup dry bread crumbs
1 tablespoon ground pecans

Wash the spinach in cold water to remove any grit. Cook in a large pot with just the water left clinging to the leaves until wilted. Let cool and squeeze all liquid from the leaves. Transfer to a food processor. Chop with on/off turns.

Add the egg substitute, yogurt, cheese, garlic, oregano, and cinnamon. In a cup, combine the bread crumbs and pecans.

Coat a 9-inch pie plate with nonstick spray. Add the bread crumb mixture and distribute evenly in the bottom and up the sides.

Pour the spinach mixture into the pan. Bake at 400°F for 30 to 40 minutes, or until a knife inserted in the center comes out clean.

Serves 4

ONION AND PESTO PIE

◇ *Per serving*

119 calories
2.8 g. fat
(21% of calories)
0.9 g. dietary fiber
5 mg. cholesterol
63 mg. sodium

2 cups thinly sliced onions
1 tablespoon olive oil
3 cups nonfat cottage cheese
3 cloves garlic, chopped

2 tablespoons minced fresh parsley
1 teaspoon dried basil
2 tablespoons lemon juice
½ cup egg substitute

¼ cup grated Sapsago or Parmesan cheese
¼ teaspoon grated nutmeg
⅛ teaspoon black pepper

*I*n a large nonstick frying pan over medium heat, sauté the onions in 1 teaspoon of the oil until soft, about 10 minutes. Cool.

In a food processor, blend the cottage cheese, garlic, parsley, and basil with on/off turns until well combined. With the motor running, gradually add the lemon juice and the remaining oil. Transfer to a large bowl.

Add the onions, egg substitute, cheese, nutmeg, and pepper. Mix well.

Coat a 9-inch springform pan with nonstick spray. Pour in the onion mixture. Bake at 350°F for 45 to 60 minutes, or until a knife inserted in the center comes out clean. Let cool on a wire rack for 20 minutes. Remove the sides of the pan.

Serves 6

◇   ◇   ◇

GREEK SPINACH AND RICE

◇ *Per serving*

273 calories
3.7 g. fat
(12% of calories)
6.2 g. dietary fiber
6 mg. cholesterol
369 mg. sodium

1 cup minced onions
2 tablespoons defatted stock
1 pound spinach, chopped
3 cups cold cooked rice

1 cup low-fat cottage cheese
¼ cup shredded low-fat Cheddar cheese

¼ cup egg substitute
3 tablespoons minced fresh parsley
1½ teaspoons dillweed

*I*n a large nonstick frying pan, cook the onions in the stock until soft. Add the spinach and cook over low heat, stirring constantly, until wilted. Cook until all liquid has evaporated.

In a large bowl, combine the rice, cottage cheese, Cheddar, egg substitute, parsley, and dill. Fold in the spinach mixture.

Coat a 1½-quart casserole with nonstick spray. Add the rice mixture. Bake at 375°F for 20 to 25 minutes, or until heated through and light brown on top.

Serves 4

INDONESIAN STIR-FRY

◇ *Per serving*

425 calories
11.1 g. fat
(24% of calories)
3.9 g. dietary fiber
0 mg. cholesterol
279 mg. sodium

3 hot green chili peppers, seeded and minced
2 tablespoons peeled minced gingerroot
4 cloves garlic, minced
1 tablespoon canola oil

1 cup diced sweet red peppers
1 cup thinly sliced scallions
2 cups defatted stock
3 tablespoons peanut butter
2 tablespoons low-sodium soy sauce

1 tablespoon lemon juice
1 teaspoon honey
½ teaspoon red-pepper flakes
1 cup cubed tofu
6 cups hot cooked rice

*I*n a large nonstick frying pan over medium heat, sauté the chili peppers, ginger, and garlic in the oil for 5 minutes. Add the red peppers and scallions. Stir for 1 to 2 minutes, or until the scallions are limp.

Add the stock, stirring to loosen any bits of seasonings from the bottom of the pan. Add the peanut butter, soy sauce, lemon juice, honey, and pepper flakes. Cook over medium heat, stirring constantly, until the sauce thickens and begins to simmer.

Add the tofu. Cover the pan and reduce the heat to low. Cook for 10 minutes, or until the peppers are just tender. Serve over the rice.

Serves 6

◇   ◇   ◇

GREEK GARDEN KABOBS

◇ *Per serving*

70 calories
0.5 g. fat
(6% of calories)
1.8 g. dietary fiber

1 cup nonfat yogurt
¼ cup minced fresh mint
4 cloves garlic, minced

½ teaspoon dried oregano
1 large eggplant, cut into 1½-inch chunks

20 cherry tomatoes

1 mg. cholesterol
54 mg. sodium

*I*n a shallow baking dish, combine ½ cup yogurt, 2 tablespoons mint, half of the garlic, and a pinch of oregano.

Add the eggplant and toss to coat well. Cover and allow to marinate for 30 mintues.

Thread the eggplant and tomatoes onto skewers. Broil or grill about 4 inches from the heat for about 2 minutes on each side.

In a small bowl, combine the remaining yogurt, mint, garlic, and oregano. Use as a dipping sauce for the kabobs.

Serves 4

◇   ◇   ◇

EGGS WITH CHILI SAUCE

◇ *Per serving*

228 calories
5.6 g. fat
(22% of calories)
2.5 g. dietary fiber
1 mg. cholesterol
171 mg. sodium

1 large onion, minced
3 cloves garlic, minced
1 tablespoon olive oil
1½ cups shredded romaine lettuce

3 hot or mild chili peppers, chopped
¼ cup chopped fresh coriander
½ teaspoon dried oregano
1½ cups egg substitute

4 flour tortillas
1 avocado, thinly sliced (optional)
1 cup nonfat yogurt
1 cup alfalfa sprouts
1 cup diced tomatoes

*I*n a large nonstick frying pan, cook the onions and garlic in the oil until limp. Add the lettuce, chili peppers, coriander, and oregano. Cook for about 3 minutes, or until the lettuce has wilted. Transfer to a large bowl.

Clean the frying pan and coat with nonstick spray. Add the egg substitute and cook over low heat until lightly scrambled.

Divide among the tortillas. Top with the chili mixture. Do not roll the tortillas. Serve flat topped with the avocados (if using), yogurt, sprouts, and tomatoes.

Serves 4

BROCCOLI QUESADILLA

◇ *Per serving*

185 calories
5.2 g. fat
(25% of calories)
2.9 g. dietary fiber
3 mg. cholesterol
216 mg. sodium

1 head broccoli, broken into large florets
2 teaspoons olive oil
1 red onion, finely chopped
2 cloves garlic, minced
½ teaspoon ground cumin
¼ teaspoon chili powder

⅛ teaspoon ground cinnamon
2 jalapeño peppers, seeded and minced
6 cherry tomatoes, quartered
1 tablespoon minced fresh coriander

6 flour tortillas
¼ cup shredded part-skim mozzarella cheese
1 cup salsa
1 cup nonfat yogurt
1 avocado, sliced (optional)

Steam the broccoli until crisp-tender. Chop coarsely and set aside.

In a large nonstick frying pan, heat 1 teaspoon of the oil. Add the onions and sauté over medium heat for 3 to 4 minutes to soften. Add the garlic, cumin, chili powder, and cinnamon. Cook for 1 minute.

Add the broccoli, peppers, tomatoes, and coriander. Stir well and sauté another 3 to 4 minutes. Transfer to a bowl and set aside.

Clean the frying pan. Brush lightly with some of the remaining oil and heat over medium-high heat.

Divide the broccoli mixture among the tortillas. Sprinkle with the cheese. Fold in half.

Working in batches, fry each tortilla for 2 to 3 minutes per side, pressing with a spatula to flatten it a bit. Brush the pan with more oil as necessary.

To serve, top each tortilla with salsa, yogurt, and avocados (if used).

Serves 6

POLENTA: CORNMEAL BY ANOTHER NAME

Polenta is a hearty peasant dish made from cornmeal. The Italians have relished it for centuries. Today, it's making a comeback as a filling, complex-carbohydrate dish that's a refreshing change from potatoes, rice, and noodles.

Basically, polenta is cornmeal that's cooked until thick, cooled until firm, cut into slices, and topped with a sauce. Depending on the topping, it can serve as an appetizer, a main course, or a side dish.

Although making the polenta itself takes a bit of time, you can do that part at your leisure. For that matter, you can prepare the topping ahead of time, too. Then it's a simple matter of reheating the two for dinner in a flash.

◇ ────────────────────

Polenta

1 cup yellow cornmeal	2½ cups defatted stock	1½ teaspoons olive oil
1 cup water		

In a large bowl, whisk together the cornmeal and water.

In a 3-quart saucepan, bring the stock and oil to a boil. Whisk in the cornmeal and stir until the mixture thickens, about 3 or 4 minutes. That will keep the polenta smooth and free of lumps.

Cook over medium heat, stirring constantly with a wooden spoon, for 25 minutes.

Cover the pot and leave it on the heat for 3 minutes, without stirring. Shake the pot a little to allow some steam to get under the polenta so it will unmold from the pot easily.

Coat an 8½ × 4½-inch loaf pan with nonstick spray. Add the polenta and allow to set until quite firm.

Unmold it onto a cutting board or countertop. Cut into ¾- to 1-inch slices.

Sauté, broil, or bake the slices until hot, then add your choice of topping.

Serves 4

◇*Per serving: 148 calories, 3.7 g. fat (23% of calories), 4.7 g. dietary fiber, 0 mg. cholesterol, 63 mg. sodium*

(continued)

Mediterranean Topping

1 cup sliced onions

1½ teaspoons olive oil

2 cups broccoli florets

1½ cups sliced mushrooms

1 cup sliced yellow summer squash

1 cup crushed tomatoes

¼ cup minced fresh coriander

½ teaspoon dried savory

¼ teaspoon dried thyme

¼ teaspoon hot-pepper sauce

Polenta (page 169)

In a large frying pan over medium heat, sauté the onions in the oil until soft, about 5 minutes. Add the broccoli, mushrooms, and squash. Sauté for 5 minutes.

Add the tomatoes, coriander, savory, thyme, and hot-pepper sauce.

Cover and cook 20 minutes, or until the vegetables are tender. Serve over the polenta.

Serves 4

◇*Per serving:* 213 calories, 5.7 g. fat (24% of calories), 7.7 g. dietary fiber, 0 mg. cholesterol, 132 mg. sodium

◇ ──────────────────────────

Primavera Sauce

1 cup julienned carrots

1 cup julienned zucchini

½ cup julienned scallions

3 tablespoons unbleached flour

1½ cups skim milk

1 teaspoon Dijon mustard

1 teaspoon dillweed

Polenta (page 169)

Steam the carrots, zucchini, and scallions until tender, about 4 minutes.

In a 2-quart saucepan, combine the flour and ¼ cup of the milk. Whisk until smooth. Whisk in the remaining milk. Cook, whisking constantly, until the sauce thickens and comes to a boil. Whisk in the mustard and dill. Remove from the heat.

Stir in the vegetables. Serve over the polenta.

Serves 4

◇*Per serving:* 223 calories, 4.1 g. fat (17% of calories), 6.5 g. dietary fiber, 2 mg. cholesterol, 148 mg. sodium

◇ ─────────────────────────────

Asparagus Topping

2 cups sliced asparagus
1 cup sliced mushrooms
½ cup minced shallots
2 tablespoons defatted stock
1 teaspoon olive oil
2 teaspoons snipped chives
½ teaspoon dried tarragon
¼ cup shredded low-fat Colby cheese
Polenta (page 169)

Steam the asparagus until tender, about 5 to 7 minutes.

In a large frying pan, combine the mushrooms, shallots, stock, and oil. Cook over medium heat until the mushrooms are tender. Stir in the chives, tarragon, and asparagus. Heat through. Sprinkle with the cheese. Serve over the polenta.

Serves 4

◇*Per serving:* 218 calories, 6 g. fat (25% of calories), 6 g. dietary fiber, 2 mg. cholesterol, 91 mg. sodium

SPICY VEGETABLES WITH TOFU

1 onion, thinly sliced
1 sweet red pepper, cut into 2-inch strips
2 stalks celery, thinly sliced diagonally
4 cloves garlic, minced
1 tablespoon peeled minced gingerroot

1 tablespoon minced chili pepper
1 tablespoon canola oil
¼ cup thinly sliced mushrooms
¾ cup broccoli florets
¾ cup sliced cauliflower florets

¼ cup peas
1 cup cubed tofu
¼ cup defatted stock
1 tablespoon low-sodium soy sauce
4 cups hot cooked rice

*I*n a large frying pan over medium heat, sauté the onions, red peppers, celery, garlic, ginger, and chili peppers in the oil for 5 minutes. Add the mushrooms, broccoli, cauliflower, and peas. Stir to combine.

Add the tofu, stock, and soy sauce. Cover and cook for 3 to 4 minutes, or until the vegetables are crisp-tender.

Serve over the rice.

Serves 4

ITALIAN-STYLE FRIED RICE

8 artichoke hearts, chopped
1 cup thinly sliced onions
2 cloves garlic, minced

1 shallot, minced
3 tablespoons olive oil
2 cups shredded spinach
4 cups cold cooked rice

3 tablespoons grated Sapsago or Parmesan cheese

*I*n a large nonstick frying pan, sauté the artichokes, onions, garlic, and shallots in 1 tablespoon of the oil until tender, about 4 minutes.

Add the spinach and sauté until the spinach wilts. Transfer to a large bowl.

Sauté the rice in the remaining oil until heated through. Stir in the spinach mixture. Sprinkle with the cheese.

Serves 4

◇　　　　　　　　　　　◇　　　　　　　　　　　◇

SPICY STUFFED PEPPERS

◇ *Per serving*

191 calories
5.2 g. fat
(25% of calories)
6.3 g. dietary fiber
0 mg. cholesterol
22 mg. sodium

⅓ cup minced
   scallions
1 clove garlic,
   minced
1 tablespoon
   olive oil
2 tomatoes,
   chopped
1 jalapeño
   pepper,
   seeded and
   thinly sliced

2 tablespoons
   minced fresh
   parsley
1 teaspoon
   dried oregano
1 teaspoon
   ground cumin

1 bay leaf
2 cups corn
1 cup cooked
   black beans
4 large sweet
   red peppers

*I*n a large frying pan, cook the scallions and garlic in the oil until soft, about 4 minutes. Add the tomatoes, jalapeño peppers, parsley, oregano, cumin, and bay leaf. Bring to a boil and cook, stirring frequently, until the tomatoes are soft and the mixture has thickened, about 10 minutes.

Add the corn, partially cover, and simmer about 8 minutes. Discard the bay leaf. Stir in the beans. Keep warm over very low heat.

Cut about ½ inch off the top of each pepper. Discard the seeds. Steam the whole peppers until tender.

Divide the stuffing among the peppers.

Serves 4

Potato Bake with Mushroom Stroganoff

◇ *Per serving*

249 calories
4.5 g. fat
(16% of calories)
5.9 g. dietary fiber
2 mg. cholesterol
107 mg. sodium

4	large baking potatoes	2	cloves garlic, minced
1½	cups nonfat yogurt	1	tablespoon olive oil
1	teaspoon Dijon mustard	1½	pounds small mushrooms, quartered
1	large onion, diced		

½ teaspoon dillweed

½ teaspoon dried thyme

⅛ teaspoon grated nutmeg

*B*ake the potatoes at 375°F for 1 hour, or until easily pierced with a fork.

While the potatoes are baking, line a strainer with cheesecloth and set it over a bowl. Add the yogurt and set it aside to drain for about 15 minutes. Transfer to a small bowl. Whisk in the mustard and set aside.

In a large nonstick frying pan over medium-high heat, sauté the onions and garlic in the oil until the onions wilt, about 5 minutes.

Add the mushrooms, dill, thyme, and nutmeg. Sauté until the mushrooms are brown and fragrant, about 10 minutes. Remove from the heat.

Stir in the yogurt mixture.

Serve over the potatoes.

Serves 4

MEXICAN CORN CASSEROLE

◇ *Per serving*

282 calories
5.8 g. fat
(19% of calories)
9.1 g. dietary fiber
9 mg. cholesterol
351 mg. sodium

1 cup minced onions
½ cup minced green peppers
3 cloves garlic, minced
2 tablespoons water
2 cups chopped tomatoes
¼ cup minced fresh coriander

¾ teaspoon dried oregano
½ teaspoon ground cumin
2 teaspoons red-wine vinegar
2½ cups defatted stock
1 cup cornmeal

2 cups corn
½ cup shredded low-fat Monterey Jack cheese
½ cup chopped mild chili peppers
½ cup minced scallions

*I*n a large frying pan, sauté the onions, green peppers, and garlic in the water until tender, about 5 minutes. Add the tomatoes, coriander, oregano, and cumin. Bring to a boil. Cover, reduce the heat, and simmer 10 minutes. Remove the lid and cook, stirring, until thick. Stir in the vinegar.

Place the stock in a 2-quart saucepan. Whisk in the cornmeal. Cook over medium heat, stirring constantly, until the mixture bubbles and becomes very thick, about 15 minutes. Stir in the corn.

Coat a 9-inch pie plate with nonstick spray. Spread half of the corn filling in the plate. Sprinkle with the cheese, chili peppers, and scallions. Cover with the remaining corn mixture. Top with the tomato mixture.

Bake at 350°F for 40 minutes.

Serves 4

CORN ENCHILADAS

◇ *Per serving*

355 calories
6.6 g. fat
(17% of calories)
5.1 g. dietary fiber
6 mg. cholesterol
79 mg. sodium

1 large dried chili pepper (preferably ancho)
2 teaspoons canola oil
1 cup corn
½ cup minced sweet red peppers
2 scallions, minced
2 cloves garlic, minced

1½ cups cold cooked rice
½ teaspoon dried oregano
½ teaspoon hot-pepper sauce
¼ teaspoon ground cinnamon
¼ cup shredded low-fat cheese

4 flour tortillas
2 tablespoons lime juice
1 cup nonfat yogurt
¼ cup minced fresh coriander
2 cups orange sections

*P*lace the chili pepper in a small bowl and cover with boiling water. Let stand until softened, about 15 minutes. Discard the stem and seeds. Mince the pepper; reserve the soaking water.

In a large nonstick frying pan, heat the oil. Add the chili peppers, corn, red peppers, scallions, and garlic. Sauté about 5 minutes.

Add the rice, oregano, hot-pepper sauce, and cinnamon. Sauté for several minutes, until heated through. Remove from the heat and stir in the cheese.

Reserve about ½ cup of filling. Divide the remainder among the tortillas. Roll up each tortilla to enclose the filling.

In the same frying pan, heat the lime juice and ½ cup of the reserved soaking liquid. Place the tortillas in the pan, seam-side down. Cover and simmer until the liquid has been absorbed and the enchiladas are heated through, about 5 minutes.

In a small bowl, combine the yogurt and coriander.

Serve the enchiladas topped with reserved filling, yogurt, and orange sections.

Serves 4

EGGS: THE REAL THING?

You may notice that most of the recipes in this book call for egg whites or egg substitute rather than whole eggs. That's because most people would prefer to limit their cholesterol intake. And egg yolks are particularly rich in cholesterol—the usual estimate is 250 to 275 milligrams in a single large yolk. For people on a strict cholesterol-lowering diet, that's almost twice their cholesterol quota for an entire day.

Egg whites, on the other hand, are composed almost entirely of low-cal, high-quality protein. So you can eat all you want. Egg substitutes are made mostly of egg whites and contain no cholesterol and fewer calories than whole eggs. Some brands have no fat at all; others weigh in at about half of what's in an egg. Read the labels.

Here are some tips for using egg substitutes and egg whites.

- Thaw egg substitute before using and store leftovers in the refrigerator. Use the excess within a week.
- For casseroles and most baked goods, replace each whole egg with 2 egg whites or ¼ cup egg substitute.
- In dishes where only egg yolks are required, use ¼ cup egg substitute for each yolk. But be aware that recipes calling for more than 2 yolks may not turn out well if made with egg sub.
- When making cakes, get nice volume by increasing the egg substitute to ⅓ cup in place of each whole egg.
- If making a cake that calls for three or four eggs, reduce the amount of liquid (usually milk) by 2 tablespoons to compensate for the extra egg liquid.
- Because egg substitute is pasteurized, it's suitable for uncooked salad dressings and mayonnaise.
- Egg substitutes do contain real egg, so treat foods you prepare with them just as you would egg dishes. Refrigerate custards, mayonnaise-based salads, and other foods as usual.
- You can make omelets, frittatas, and scrambled eggs with all whites. Add a little mustard for egg-yolk color.
- For reduced-cholesterol egg dishes, pair one yolk with two, three, or four whites.

Spaghetti Squash with Tomato Sauce

◇ *Per serving*

140 calories
3.1 g. fat
(20% of calories)
10.8 g. dietary fiber
4 mg. cholesterol
139 mg. sodium

1 large spaghetti squash
1 large onion, diced
2 cloves garlic, minced

5 plum tomatoes, chopped
½ cup tomato puree
1 teaspoon dried oregano

½ teaspoon black pepper
3 tablespoons grated Parmesan cheese

*P*lace the squash in a very large pot. Add water to cover. Bring to a boil and cook, uncovered, for 30 to 60 minutes, or until easily pierced with a fork. Drain, halve, and set aside until cool enough to handle.

Coat a 2-quart saucepan with nonstick spray. Add the onions and sauté over medium heat until translucent, about 5 minutes. Add the garlic and sauté 1 minute.

Add the tomatoes, tomato puree, oregano, and pepper. Simmer for 20 minutes.

Discard the seeds from the squash. Using a fork, separate the flesh into spaghetti-like strands. Reheat briefly in a large frying pan. Serve topped with the sauce and sprinkled with the cheese.

Serves 4

◇   ◇   ◇

Enchiladas with Cheese and Kale

◇ *Per serving*

289 calories
7.9 g. fat
(25% of calories)
6.7 g. dietary fiber

2 cups shredded kale
½ cup minced scallions
2 teaspoons olive oil

8 corn tortillas
1 cup shredded low-fat Monterey Jack cheese

1 cup cooked pinto beans
1 cup salsa

vegetarian main meals

5 mg. cholesterol
372 mg. sodium

*I*n a large nonstick frying pan over medium heat, sauté the kale and scallions in 1 teaspoon of the oil until tender, about 5 minutes.

Divide the mixture among the tortillas. Top with the cheese and beans. Roll up each tortilla to enclose the filling.

Clean the frying pan and warm it over medium heat. Add the remaining oil. Place the enchiladas, seam-side down, in the pan. Let brown for several minutes on each side.

Add the salsa. Cover the pan, reduce the heat, and simmer for about 5 minutes, basting frequently.

Serves 4

◇   ◇   ◇

VEGETABLE PAELLA

◇ *Per serving*

271 calories
4.5 g. fat
(15% of calories)
4.5 g. dietary fiber
0 mg. cholesterol
49 mg. sodium

¼ cup defatted stock
1 teaspoon turmeric
1 sweet red pepper, thinly sliced
4 Italian tomatoes, diced

2 medium zucchini, thinly sliced
3 cups cold cooked rice
1 tablespoon olive oil
2 tablespoons grated Sapsago or Parmesan cheese

2 tablespoons minced fresh parsley

*I*n a large nonstick frying pan, combine the stock and turmeric. Add the peppers, tomatoes, and zucchini. Cook until the vegetables are crisp-tender, about 5 minutes. Transfer to a large bowl.

Add the rice and oil to the pan. Stir-fry over medium-high heat for 5 minutes. Add the vegetables and stir to combine. Sprinkle with the cheese and parsley.

Serves 4

CHAPTER NINE ◇

Fish and Seafood

U ntil a few years ago, fish was considered "health food" because of what it didn't have—lots of fat and calories. Dieters ordered fish as a lean alternative to steak, chops, and other red meats. Then scientists stumbled across an intriguing phenomenon: Heart disease was rare among Greenland Eskimos, despite their high consumption of animal fats (including whale blubber). But the Eskimos also ate a lot of fatty fish such as mackerel, and therein lies the clue to this dietary paradox.

Mackerel happens to be the richest source of special polyunsaturated fats called omega-3 fatty acids. These fatty acids, also found in other deep-water fish such as salmon and tuna, may help lower blood levels of cholesterol. In some studies, they inhibited the formation of plaque on artery walls, fending off heart disease and stroke.

What's more, shellfish—mollusks and crustaceans such as shrimp, crab, oysters, and clams—also contain omega-3's. And seafood in general tends to be high in important minerals. Clams, for example, are a tremendous source of blood-building iron, and oysters are loaded with zinc for fighting off infections.

The only catch? To benefit from the healing powers of fish, you should probably eat two or three sea meals a week. But with recipes like the ones in this chapter, that shouldn't be too hard to swallow. Dark-fleshed fish such as salmon and mackerel are your best bets, but even milder varieties contribute health-building omega-3's. So eat hearty, matey.

Swordfish and Pineapple Brochettes

◇ *Per serving*

216 calories
5.1 g. fat
(21% of calories)
1.6 g. dietary fiber
44 mg. cholesterol
246 mg. sodium

1 small
  pineapple
⅓ cup orange
  juice
¼ cup peeled
  chopped
  gingerroot

1 pound
  swordfish
  steaks, 1 inch
  thick
3 tablespoons
  nonfat
  mayonnaise

*P*eel and core the pineapple. Cut part of the flesh into 12 (1-inch) cubes and reserve.

Coarsely chop the best of the pineapple and place in a blender. Add the orange juice and ginger. Puree. Pour into a bowl or shallow baking dish.

Cut the swordfish into 16 cubes. Add to the pineapple mixture, toss to coat, cover, and allow to marinate in the refrigerator for 1 hour.

For each serving, alternate four swordfish cubes and three pineapple cubes on an 8-inch skewer. Reserve the marinade.

Place the skewers on a lightly oiled broiler pan. Broil about 4 inches from the heat for 4 to 5 minutes, turning three times to evenly broil all sides.

Place the reserved marinade in a 1-quart saucepan. Bring to a boil. Pour into a bowl. Whisk in the mayonnaise until smooth. Serve with the brochettes.

Serves 4

Monkfish with Citrus and Ginger

◇ *Per serving*

390 calories
9.5 g. fat
(22% of calories)
5.8 g. dietary fiber
35 mg. cholesterol
34 mg. sodium

1¼ pounds monkfish fillets
2 tablespoons olive oil
2 cloves garlic, minced
3 cups sugar snap peas
2 scallions, sliced
1 tablespoon peeled minced gingerroot
1 tablespoon grated orange rind
2 cups orange sections
2 cups hot cooked rice

*T*rim the membrane and any discolored areas from the fish. Cut the fish diagonally into 2-inch by ½-inch strips.

In a large nonstick frying pan over medium-high heat, heat 1 tablespoon of oil. Add half of the fish and the garlic. Sauté until the fish turns white. Remove the fish with a slotted spoon.

Add the remaining fish to the pan and sauté until white. Remove from the pan. Drain off the liquid.

In the same pan, heat the remaining 1 tablespoon of oil. Add the peas, scallions, ginger, and orange rind. Cook, stirring frequently, until the peas are tender-crisp, about 6 to 8 minutes. Add the oranges and heat 1 minute.

Return the fish to the pan and heat through. Serve with the rice.

Serves 4

◇　　　　　　　　◇　　　　　　　　◇

Thyme-Flavored Tuna Steaks

◇ *Per serving*

160 calories
4.2 g. fat

2½ teaspoons olive oil
1 teaspoon dried thyme
¼ cup defatted chicken stock
1 pound tuna steaks
2 sweet red peppers, thinly sliced

(24% of calories)
0.6 g. dietary fiber
51 mg. cholesterol
48 mg. sodium

*I*n a small bowl, combine the oil, thyme, and stock. Rub on both sides of each piece of fish.

Place the tuna in a single layer in a glass baking dish. Cover with the red peppers. Drizzle with any remaining oil mixture.

Bake at 350°F for 30 to 45 minutes, or until the fish flakes easily with a fork.

Serves 4

◇ ◇ ◇

CHINESE BRAISED MACKEREL

◇ *Per serving*

464 calories
12.8 g. fat
(25% of calories)
2.9 g. dietary fiber
59 mg. cholesterol
135 mg. sodium

¼ cup rice-wine vinegar
½ teaspoon low-sodium soy sauce
3 thin slices peeled gingerroot, julienned

3 cloves garlic, minced
12 ounces mackerel fillets
1 cup defatted chicken stock

3 white icicle radishes, julienned
1 large carrot, julienned
5 scallions, julienned
4 cups hot cooked rice

*I*n a glass baking dish, combine the vinegar, soy sauce, ginger, and garlic. Add the mackerel, skin-side up, in a single layer. Marinate for at least 10 minutes.

In a large nonstick frying pan, bring the stock to a boil. Reduce the heat to a simmer. Add the mackerel, skin-side up, and the marinade. Cover and simmer 5 minutes.

Add the radishes and carrots. Simmer 2 to 3 minutes. With a slotted spoon, transfer the mackerel and vegetables to a serving platter.

Boil the liquid until reduced by half. Pour over the fish. Sprinkle with the scallions. Serve over the rice.

Serves 4

GREAT GRILLING: FISH

Want a low-fat, brimming-with-nutrients alternative to hot dogs, burgers, and barbecued chicken? Fish is made to order. For the best results:

■ Use firm-fleshed fish, such as catfish, grouper, halibut, marlin, monkfish, red snapper, rockfish, sablefish, salmon, shark, swordfish, tilefish, or tuna.

■ Make sure fillets and steaks are at least 1 inch thick so they're less likely to fall apart on the grill.

■ Marinate the fish before grilling. Try a mixture of 2 tablespoons lime juice and 1 tablespoon canola oil. Add herbs to taste. Cover and let stand in the refrigerator for about 30 minutes.

■ Coat the grilling rack with nonstick spray. Heat it until very hot.

■ Place the fish on the hot rack and cover with a lid. Cook 3 to 4 minutes. Use a spatula to reposition the fish at a 45-degree angle to its original placement (don't flip it, or it may fall apart). Cover and cook 3 to 4 minutes. Don't overcook.

■ For a no-cleanup fish dish, try the following succulent combination.

◇ ───────────────────────────

Fish in Foil

4 ounces firm fish	1 parsley sprig
1 thin onion slice, separated into rings	Pinch of paprika
2 thin green pepper rings	Pinch of ground white pepper
2 thin lemon slices	2 teaspoons lemon juice

Place the fish on a 12 × 14-inch piece of foil. Top with the onions, green peppers, lemons, parsley, paprika, and white pepper. Sprinkle with the lemon juice.

Fold the foil into an envelope around the fish to seal in the juice. Cook on an outdoor grill with the lid closed (or in a 450° F oven) for 15 to 20 minutes, or until the fish flakes easily with a fork.

Serves 1

◇*Per serving:* 118 calories, 2.7 g. fat (21% of calories), 0.4 g. dietary fiber, 0 mg. cholesterol, 61 mg. sodium

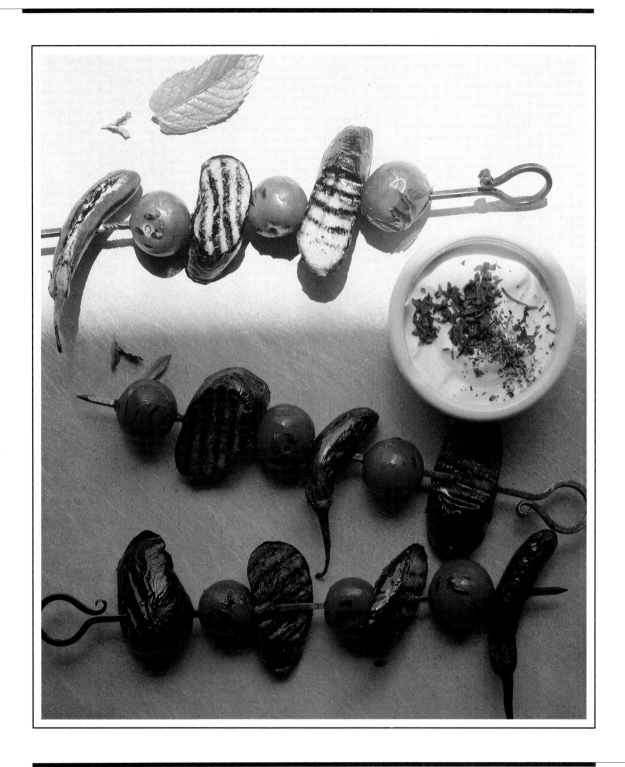

GREEK GARDEN KABOBS (PAGE 166)   185

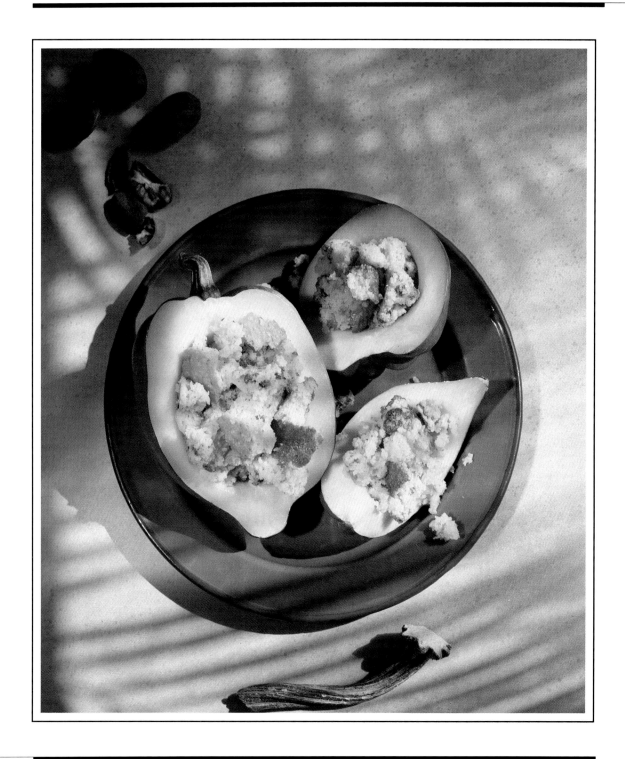

ACORN SQUASH STUFFED WITH CORNBREAD (PAGE 163)

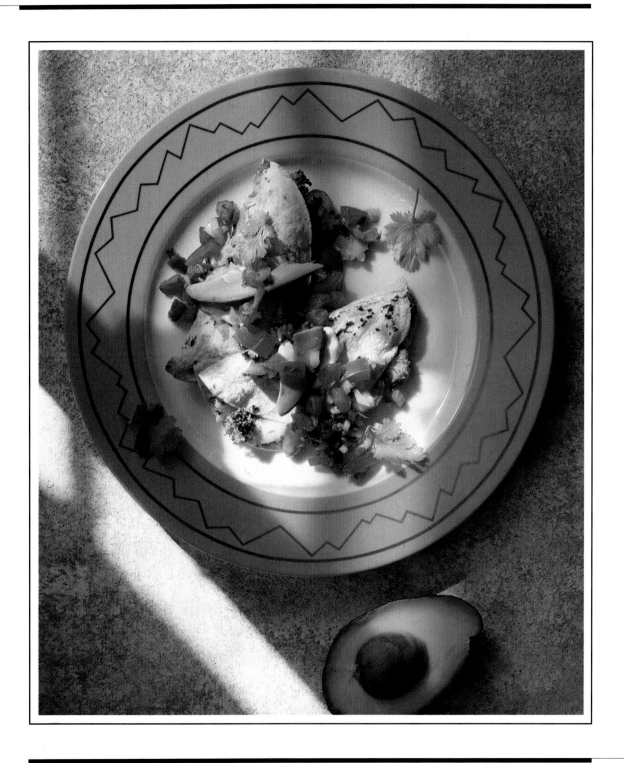

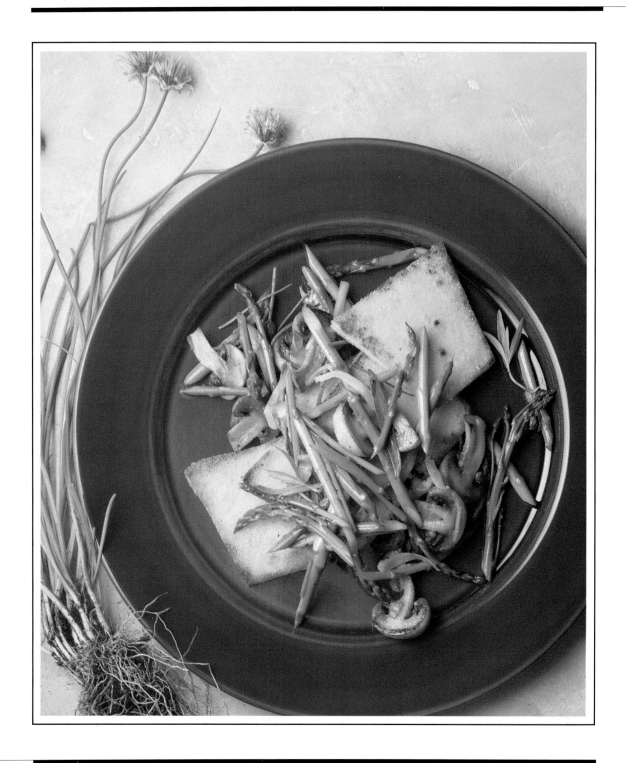

188   POLENTA (PAGE 169) WITH ASPARAGUS TOPPING (PAGE 171)

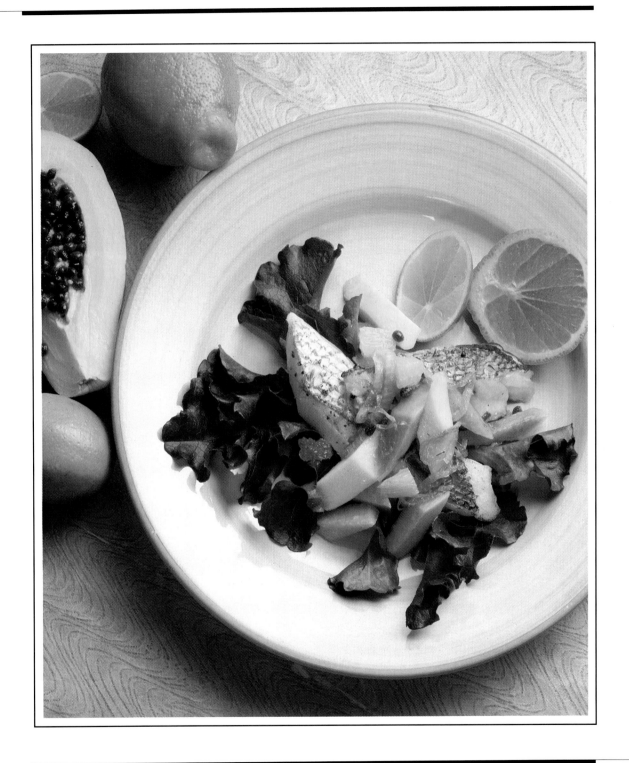

GRILLED FLORIDA SNAPPER (PAGE 204)

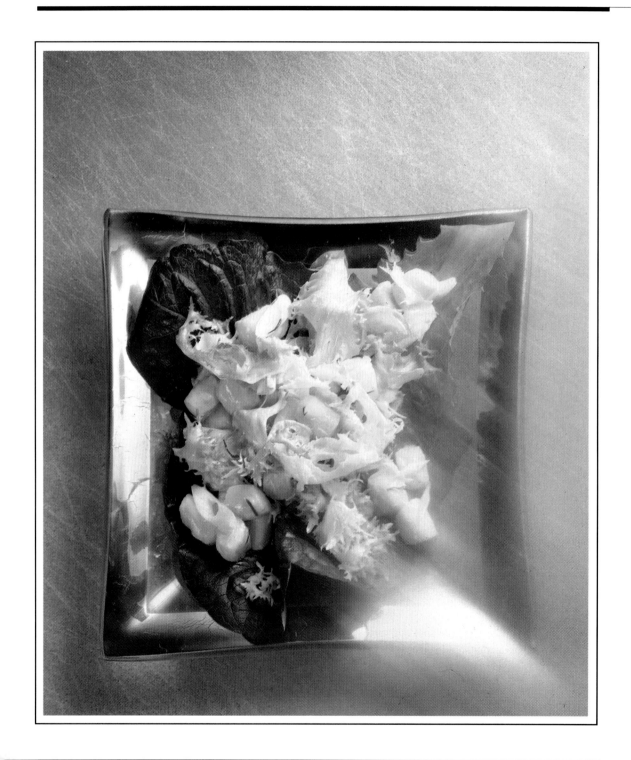

BAY SCALLOPS WITH SAFFRON (PAGE 205)

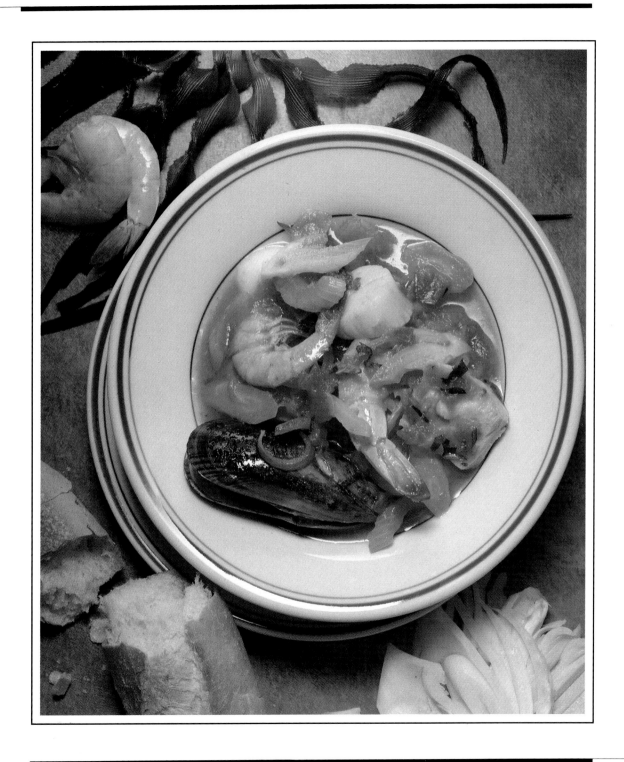

BOUILLABAISSE (PAGE 208)

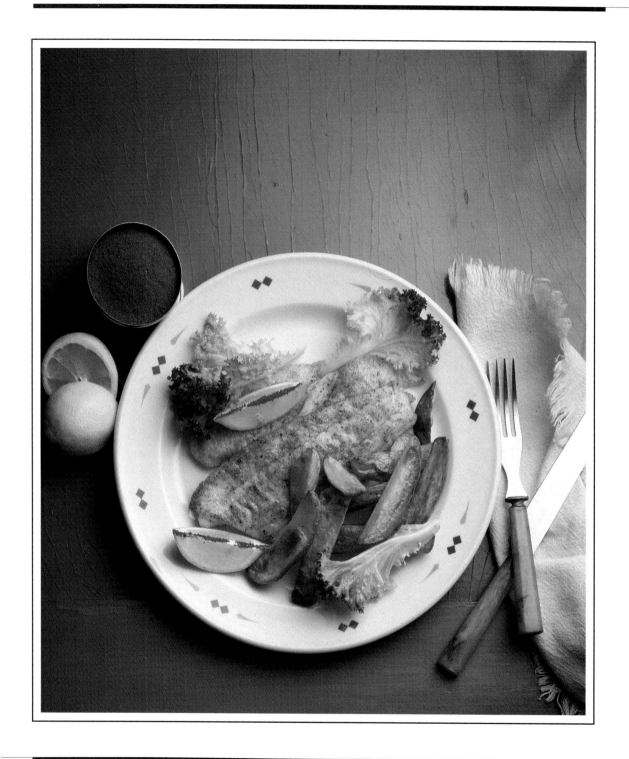

FISH AND CHIPS (PAGE 201)

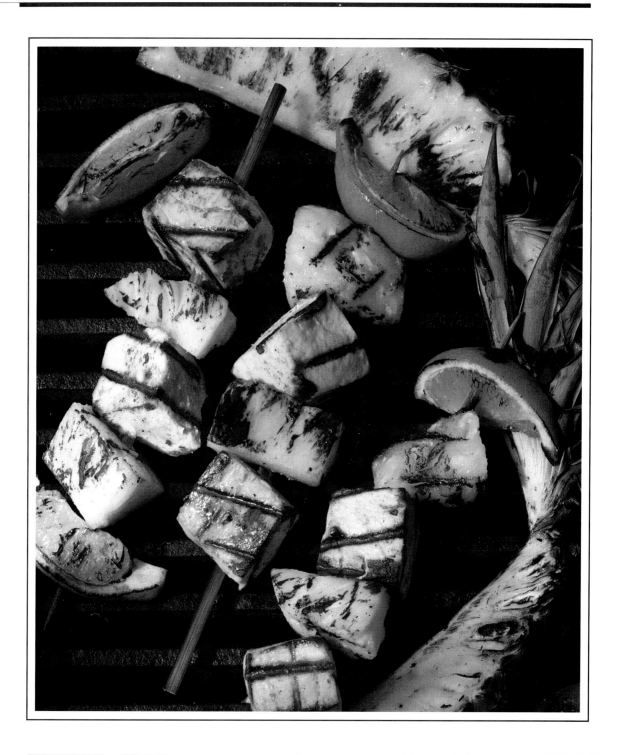

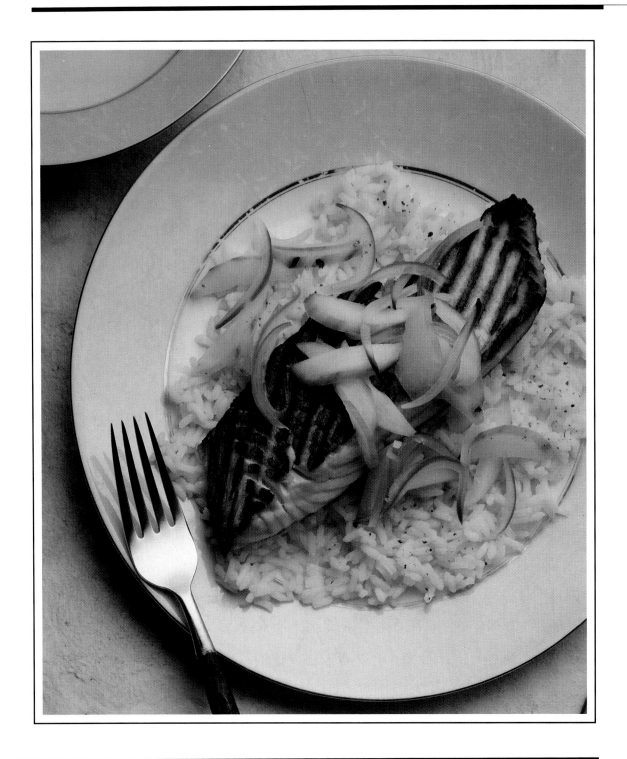

Broiled Salmon with Cucumbers (page 210)

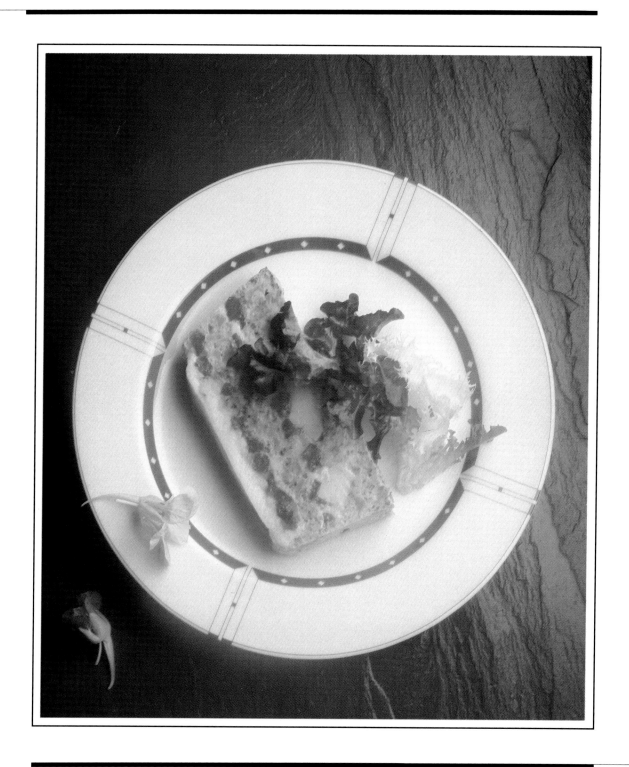

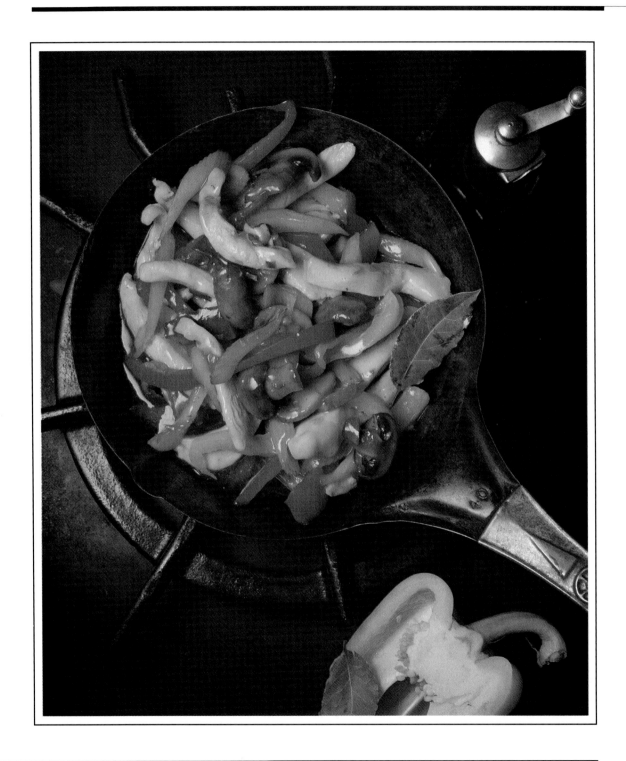

JAMAICAN CHICKEN (PAGE 232)

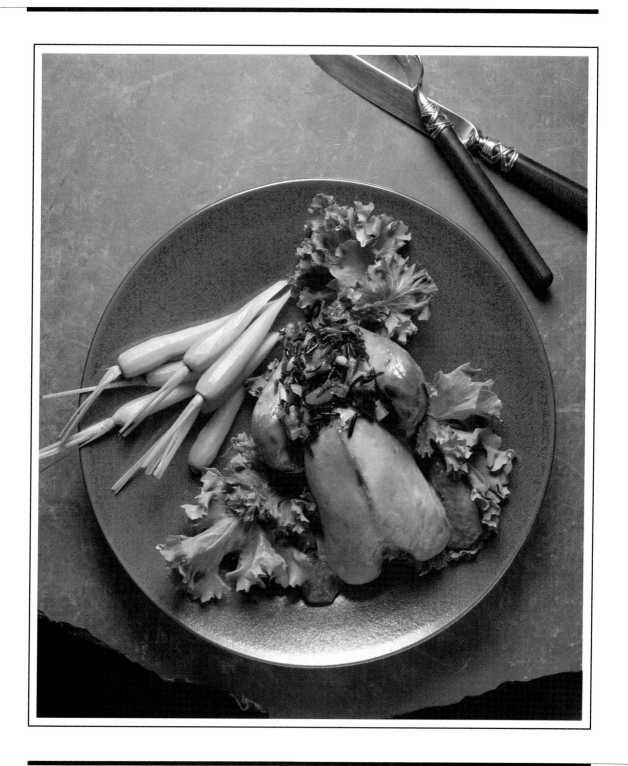

APRICOT-STUFFED HENS (PAGE 217)

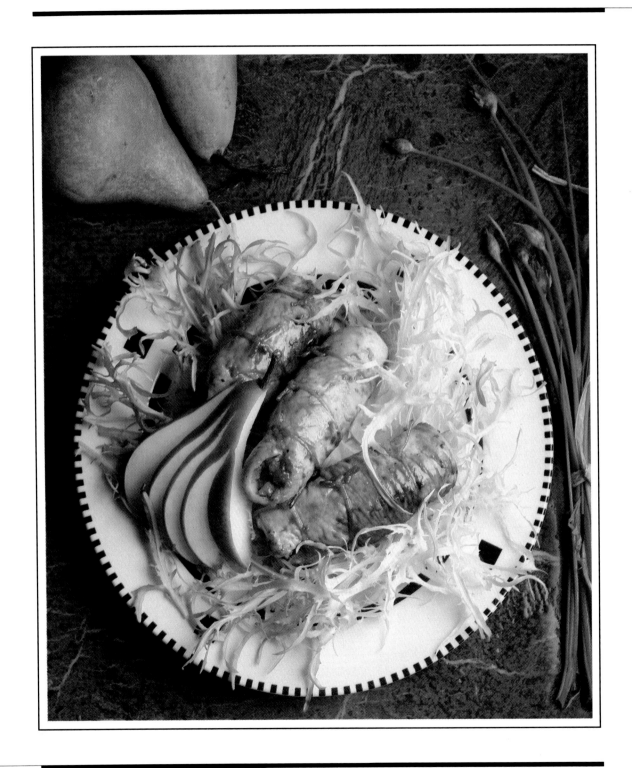

TURKEY CUTLETS WITH PEAR-PECAN STUFFING (PAGE 218)

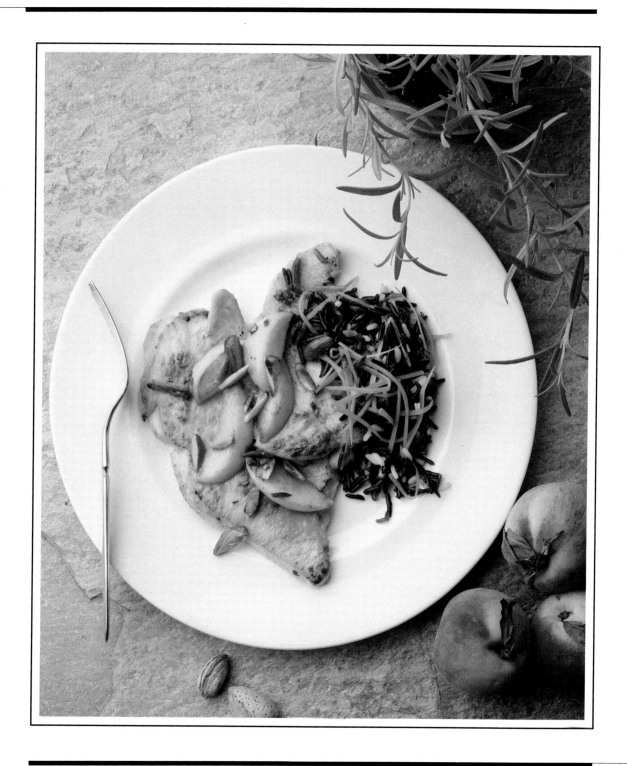

TURKEY MEDALLIONS WITH PEACHES (PAGE 252)

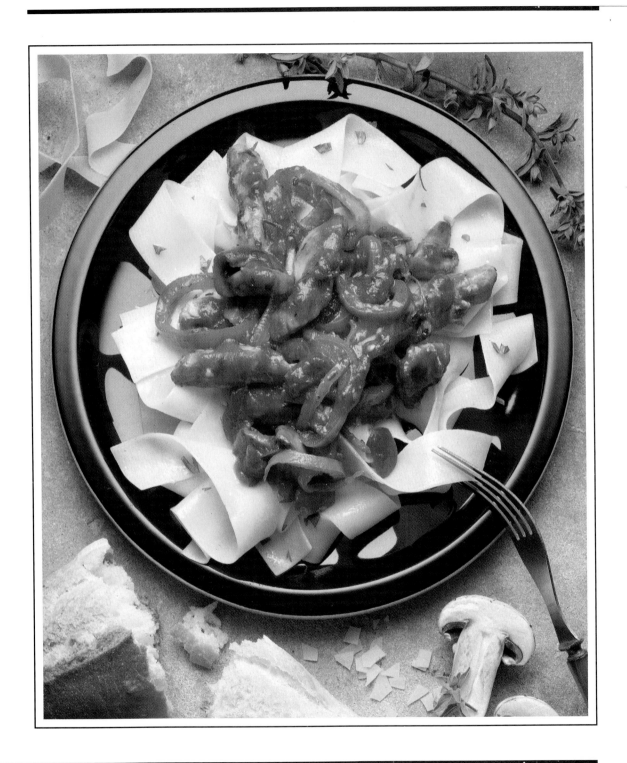

TURKEY CACCIATORE (PAGE 251)

FISH AND CHIPS

◇ *Per serving*

266 calories
7.3 g. fat
(25% of calories)
3.2 g. dietary fiber
55 mg. cholesterol
101 mg. sodium

12 small red potatoes
5 teaspoons olive oil
1 pound flounder fillets

¼ cup whole wheat flour
⅛ teaspoon red pepper

¼ cup lemon juice
½ teaspoon paprika

Scrub the potatoes, then dry thoroughly. Leaving the skins on, cut them into strips roughly 2 inches long and ½ inch thick and wide. Pat dry again.

Coat a jelly-roll pan with nonstick spray. Add the potatoes. Drizzle with 2 teaspoons of the oil. Toss to coat well.

Bake at 450°F for 30 minutes, turning the potatoes frequently.

Meanwhile, pat the fish dry. Place the flour and red pepper in a plastic bag. Add the fish, a piece at a time, and shake well to coat lightly with flour. Fold each fillet in half or roll lengthwise so all the fish can later fit in a single layer in a large frying pan.

After the potatoes have been in the oven for 30 minutes, heat a large cast-iron frying pan or other heavy, ovenproof pan over medium-high heat until quite hot. Add the remaining oil. Add the fish to the pan in a single layer. Immediately tilt the pan so you can spoon some of the oil over the fish.

Transfer the pan to the oven with the potatoes. Bake both for 10 to 15 minutes (depending upon the thickness of the fillets), until the fish is cooked through and the potatoes are crisp.

Remove the fish and potatoes from the oven. Transfer to a serving platter. Add the lemon juice to the fish pan. Stir to loosen any browned bits from the bottom. Pour over the fish. Sprinkle with the paprika.

Serves 4

Seafood-Broccoli Terrine

◇ *Per serving*

143 calories
1.2 g. fat
(8% of calories)
2 g. dietary fiber
26 mg. cholesterol
186 mg. sodium

SCALLOP LAYER
¾ cup skim milk
½ cup egg substitute
½ cup whole wheat bread crumbs
½ teaspoon grated nutmeg
⅛ teaspoon red pepper

4 ounces scallops

BROCCOLI LAYER
¼ cup whole wheat flour
1⅓ cups skim milk
¼ cup lemon juice
½ cup egg substitute

1 tablespoon dillweed
2 cups steamed chopped broccoli

ASSEMBLY
8 ounces sole fillets
1 cup steamed diced sweet red peppers

To make the scallop layer: In a large bowl, combine the milk, egg substitute, bread crumbs, nutmeg, and red pepper. If using sea scallops, cut them into quarters; if using bay scallops, leave them whole. Fold the scallops into egg mixture. Set aside.

To make the broccoli layer: Mix the flour with about ⅓ cup milk in a 2-quart saucepan to make a paste. Gradually whisk in the remaining milk. Whisk over medium heat until the mixture thickens. Remove from the heat. Whisk in the lemon juice, egg substitute, and dill. Fold in the broccoli. Set aside.

To assemble the terrine: Coat an 8½ × 4½-inch loaf pan with nonstick spray. Cover the bottom of the pan with the fish fillets. Sprinkle with half of the peppers. Top with half of the broccoli mixture.

Sprinkle with the remaining peppers, then top with all of the scallop mixture. Cover with the remaining broccoli mixture.

Cover the pan tightly with foil. Place the pan on a wire rack inside a larger baking dish. Pour in enough hot water to come two-thirds of the way up the sides of the loaf pan.

Bake at 350°F for 1 hour. Uncover the pan and bake for 30 to 45 minutes, or until firm. Unmold and cut into slices.

Serves 6

Are you guilty of battering your fish? That's no way to treat such a healthy food! Yet batter-fried fish is extremely popular. In fact, it's one item weight watchers and health seekers miss most when they shape up their diets. Well, rejoice. Because the following no-fry batter is so close in taste and texture to the "real thing" that even long-time fans of batter-fried fish declare it *superb*.

The secret? Egg whites, skim milk, and a very light spritzing of olive oil combine to produce old-fashioned crunch without a lot of fat and calories. And this method works as well on chicken as it does on fillets such as flounder, haddock, and cod.

Batter-Dipped Fish

½ cup skim milk
4 flounder fillets (about 12 ounces)
½ cup whole wheat flour
3 egg whites, lightly beaten
½ cup bread crumbs

⅛ teaspoon paprika
⅛ teaspoon ground white pepper
1 lemon, cut into wedges

Place the milk in a shallow dish, such as a pie plate. Add the flounder and soak for 5 minutes.

Dredge the fish in the flour to coat. Then dip in the egg whites. Dredge in the bread crumbs.

Dip the fish in the egg whites again and then into the bread crumbs again.

Coat a slotted broiler pan with nonstick spray. Place the fish on the pan. Sprinkle lightly with the paprika and pepper. Spray the fish lightly with nonstick spray (preferably one flavored with olive oil).

Bake at 400° F for 12 minutes. Serve with the lemon.

Serves 4

◇*Per serving:* *171 calories, 1.6 g. fat (8% of calories), 2.1 g. dietary fiber, 41 mg. cholesterol, 156 mg. sodium*

GRILLED FLORIDA SNAPPER

◇ *Per serving*

256 calories
5.4 g. fat
(19% of calories)
2.8 g. dietary fiber
42 mg. cholesterol
127 mg. sodium

1 large onion,
  thinly sliced
1 tablespoon
  olive oil
1 pound red
  snapper fillets

1 tablespoon
  coarse
  mustard
2 cups chopped
  orange
  sections

1 cup chopped
  papayas
⅓ cup lime juice
2 tablespoons
  honey

*I*n a large nonstick frying pan over medium-high heat, sauté the onion in the oil until soft and light brown, about 8 to 10 minutes. Set aside.

While the onions are cooking, rub the snapper on both sides with the mustard. Grill or broil about 5½ inches from the heat until cooked through, about 4½ minutes on each side. Transfer to a heated serving platter. Top with the onions, oranges, and papayas. Keep warm.

Add the lime juice and honey to the frying pan. Bring to a boil over high heat and cook, stirring frequently, until reduced by half, about 3 minutes. Drizzle over the fish.

Serves 4

LOBSTER
WITH MINT VINAIGRETTE

◇ *Per serving*

156 calories
4.1 g. fat
(24% of calories)
3 g. dietary fiber
39 mg. cholesterol
268 mg. sodium

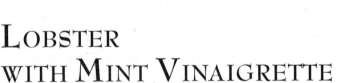

¼ cup lime
  juice
1 tablespoon
  olive oil
1 cup diced
  carrots
1 cup diced
  celery

¼ cup minced
  shallots
½ teaspoon
  dried mint
1½ cups
  chopped
  cooked
  lobster

2 papayas,
  chopped
2 cups
  shredded
  spinach

*I*n a large bowl, combine the lime juice, oil, carrots, celery, shallots, and mint. Add the lobster and papayas. Mix well. Chill. Serve the salad on the spinach.

Serves 4

◇   ◇   ◇

BAY SCALLOPS WITH SAFFRON

◇ *Per serving*

138 calories
1.2 g. fat
(8% of calories)
2.4 g. dietary fiber
37 mg. cholesterol
311 mg. sodium

¼ cup orange juice
½ teaspoon saffron
2 cloves garlic, minced
1 pound bay scallops

½ cup sliced scallions
1½ cups shredded chicory

2 tablespoons nonfat mayonnaise
1 small head red lettuce

*I*n a large nonstick frying pan over medium heat, heat the orange juice, saffron, and garlic to a simmer. Add the scallops and scallions. Sauté until the scallops are opaque, about 3 minutes.

Transfer the mixture to a large bowl. Add the chicory and mayonnaise. Toss well to combine.

Line a platter with red lettuce. Spoon the scallop mixture onto the platter. Serve warm or chilled.

Serves 4

◇   ◇   ◇

Spanish Halibut

6 tablespoons vinegar
¼ teaspoon crushed saffron
1 pound halibut fillets
1 sweet red pepper, thinly sliced

2 leeks, minced
2 cloves garlic, minced
2 teaspoons olive oil
1 teaspoon dried thyme

*I*n a large frying pan over medium heat, bring about 1 inch of water to a simmer. Stir in 4 tablespoons of the vinegar and the saffron. Add the halibut and red peppers. Simmer for 15 minutes, or until the fish flakes easily with a fork.

Use a spatula or slotted spoon to remove the fish and peppers from the liquid. Place in a 9 × 13-inch glass baking dish.

In a medium bowl, combine the remaining 2 tablespoons of vinegar with the leeks, garlic, oil, and thyme. Pour over the fish, cover, and refrigerate for at least 1 hour.

Serves 4

◇　　　　　　　　◇　　　　　　　　◇

Perch
with Mustard and Thyme

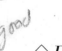
9/21/01
good

½ cup oat bran
1 pound perch fillets
2 teaspoons olive oil

½ cup defatted chicken stock
1 teaspoon Dijon mustard

½ teaspoon dried thyme

1.6 g. dietary fiber
101 mg. cholesterol
102 mg. sodium

*P*lace the oat bran on a large sheet of waxed paper. Dredge both sides of each fillet in the oat bran to coat.

Heat the oil in a nonstick frying pan. Add the fillets and sauté until cooked through, about 3½ minutes on each side.

Carefully remove the fish to a heated platter. Pour the stock into the frying pan. Whisk in the mustard and thyme. Bring to a boil and cook until reduced by half. Pour over the fish.

Serves 4

◇　　　　　　　　　◇　　　　　　　　　◇

MADRID TROUT

◇ *Per serving*

*403 calories
9.5 g. fat
(21% of calories)
4.6 g. dietary fiber
64 mg. cholesterol
94 mg. sodium*

- 1 tablespoon olive oil
- 1 cup medium-grain brown rice
- ½ cup minced celery
- ½ cup minced onions
- ½ cup minced watercress
- 3 cloves garlic, minced
- ¼ teaspoon paprika
- ¼ teaspoon dried thyme
- 2 cups defatted chicken stock
- 1 pound trout fillets
- 1 cup peeled, seeded, and chopped Italian tomatoes
- 1 cup peas

*I*n a large nonstick frying pan, heat the oil. Add the rice, celery, onions, watercress, garlic, paprika, and thyme. Stirring constantly, sauté for 3 to 4 minutes until the mixture is fragrant.

Add the stock and bring to a boil. Reduce the heat, cover, and simmer for 35 minutes, or until the rice is almost tender.

Add the fish, cover, and simmer 8 minutes. Add the tomatoes and peas. Cover and simmer for 4 minutes, or just until the peas are tender.

Serves 4

HADDOCK BLACK RAVEN

◇ *Per serving*

177 calories
4.6 g. fat
(23% of calories)
2.1 g. dietary fiber
65 mg. cholesterol
86 mg. sodium

1 tablespoon olive oil
2 onions, thinly sliced
4 cloves garlic, minced

2 cups chopped tomatoes
1 teaspoon basil vinegar
1 teaspoon dried basil

⅛ teaspoon red pepper
1 pound haddock fillets

*I*n a large nonstick frying pan over medium-low heat, heat the oil. Add the onions and garlic. Cook, stirring frequently, until soft, about 5 to 10 minutes.

Add the tomatoes, vinegar, basil, and red pepper to the pan. Cook for 10 minutes, or until most of the liquid from the tomatoes has evaporated.

Add the haddock. Cover the pan and cook until the fish is opaque and flakes easily, about 10 minutes.

Serves 4

◇ ◇ ◇

BOUILLABAISSE

◇ *Per serving*

281 calories
6.6 g. fat
(21% of calories)
3.2 g. dietary fiber
96 mg. cholesterol
426 mg. sodium

1 cup sliced carrots
1 cup sliced celery
1 cup sliced red onions
1 cup sliced fresh fennel
1 tablespoon olive oil
2 cups peeled, seeded, and chopped tomatoes

1 clove garlic, minced
¼ teaspoon saffron
2 quarts defatted stock
2 bay leaves
½ teaspoon fennel seeds
½ teaspoon dried oregano

1 pound red snapper, cut into 1-inch chunks
1 pound scallops
24 shrimp, peeled and deveined

*I*n a 4-quart pot over medium-high heat, sauté the carrots, celery, onions, and fennel in the oil for 5 minutes. Add the tomatoes, garlic, and saffron. Sauté for 5 minutes.

Add the stock, bay leaves, fennel seeds, and oregano. Bring to a boil. Reduce the heat, cover, and simmer for 30 minutes.

Add the snapper, scallops, and shrimp. Cover and simmer for 5 to 7 minutes, or until the seafood is tender. Discard the bay leaves.

Serves 6

SIZZLED SALMON WITH MINT

1 pound salmon fillet
¼ cup orange juice
2 cups chopped tomatoes

2 cups orange sections
2 tablespoons minced fresh mint

1 tablespoon olive oil
4 cups hot cooked rice

*P*lace the salmon in a baking dish. Pour the orange juice over it. Allow to marinate for about 10 minutes.

In a small bowl, combine tomatoes, oranges, and mint. Set aside.

In a large nonstick frying pan over medium-high heat, sauté the fish in the oil for about 4 minutes per side, until brown on the outside and cooked through.

Serve topped with the tomato mixture. Serve with the rice.

Serves 4

SALMON WITH SCALLIONS

◇ *Per serving*

*428 calories
11.7 g. fat
(25% of calories)
2 g. dietary fiber
62 mg. cholesterol
63 mg. sodium*

1 pound salmon fillet
1 tablespoon olive oil
¼ cup lime juice
¼ cup lemon juice

3 cloves garlic, minced
2 tablespoons minced fresh parsley
¼ teaspoon hot-pepper sauce

8 ounces linguine, cooked
½ cup minced scallions
2 large tomatoes, thinly sliced

*I*n a large nonstick frying pan over medium-high heat, sauté the salmon in the oil for 4 to 5 minutes on each side. Handle the fish gently to keep the pieces whole.

Add the lime juice, lemon juice, garlic, parsley, and hot-pepper sauce to the pan. Cook for about 3 minutes.

Transfer the salmon to a large platter. Pour the pan juices over the fish. Cover and refrigerate until chilled.

Serve over the linguine. Sprinkle with the scallions and top with the tomatoes.

Serves 4

BROILED SALMON WITH CUCUMBERS

◇ *Per serving*

*145 calories
3.8 g. fat
(24% of calories)
1.1 g. dietary fiber
24 mg. cholesterol
34 mg. sodium*

1 cup diced onions
½ cup vinegar
4 cloves garlic, minced
2 teaspoons peeled minced gingerroot

1 teaspoon low-sodium soy sauce
2 cucumbers, thinly sliced
1½ pounds salmon fillets

1 tablespoon olive oil
4 cups hot cooked rice

In a large nonstick frying pan over medium-high heat, combine the onions, vinegar, garlic, ginger, and soy sauce. Bring to a boil, stir, and cook for 3 minutes. Remove from the heat.

Add the cucumbers. Set aside to cool.

Rub the salmon on both sides with the oil. Broil about 6 inches from the heat for 4 to 5 minutes per side, or until cooked through.

Serve on a bed of rice topped with the cucumbers.

Serves 4

Bluefish in a Sea of Green

◇ *Per serving*

412 calories
11.4 g. fat
(25% of calories)
6 g. dietary fiber
100 mg. cholesterol
258 mg. sodium

¼ cup fresh bread crumbs
¼ cup thinly sliced scallions

2 tablespoons Dijon mustard
2 teaspoons olive oil
1½ pounds bluefish fillets

3 cups snow peas
1 teaspoon sesame oil
4 hot baked potatoes

In a small bowl, combine the bread crumbs, scallions, mustard, and oil.

Coat a piece of foil large enough to hold the fish in a single layer with nonstick spray. Place on a broiling pan, sprayed-side up.

Place the fish, skin-side down, on the foil. Spread with the bread crumb mixture.

Broil 8 inches from the heat for 8 to 10 minutes, or until cooked through.

In a large nonstick frying pan, stir-fry the snow peas in the sesame oil for 3 to 4 minutes, or until crisp-tender.

Arrange the peas on a platter. Top with the fish. Serve with the potatoes.

Serves 4

Herb-Steamed Mussels with Rice Pilaf

◇ *Per serving*

302 calories
6.6 g. fat
(20% of calories)
4.8 g. dietary fiber
24 mg. cholesterol
175 mg. sodium

1 tablespoon olive oil
1 cup chopped onions
3 cloves garlic, minced
1 cup long-grain white or basmati rice

1 teaspoon dried oregano
2 cups defatted chicken stock
24 mussels, scrubbed and debearded

1 large carrot, julienned
1 cup snow peas

*I*n a 14-inch paella pan (or other sloping-sided pan), heat the oil. Add the onions and garlic; sauté for 5 minutes. Add the rice and oregano; sauté for 3 minutes. Add the stock and bring to a boil. Reduce the heat and simmer for 20 minutes.

Add the mussels and carrots. Loosely cover the pan with foil. When the mussels begin to open, add the snow peas. Cover and simmer until the mussels are fully open. (The opening process should take about 6 minutes.) Discard any mussels that don't open.

Serves 4

◇   ◇

Snapper with Red-Pepper Salsa

◇ *Per serving*

218 calories
6 g. fat
(25% of calories)
1.2 g. dietary fiber

3 sweet red peppers
¼ cup minced fresh parsley
2 tablespoons minced fresh coriander

3 scallions, minced
2 tablespoons lemon juice
1 tablespoon canola oil

½ teaspoon hot-pepper sauce
1½ pounds red snapper fillets

fish and seafood

63 mg. cholesterol
115 mg. sodium

Broil the red peppers about 4 inches from the heat until blackened on all sides. Set aside until cool enough to handle. Discard the blackened skin, cores, and seeds; dice the flesh. Transfer to a medium bowl.

Add the parsley, coriander, scallions, lemon juice, oil, and hot-pepper sauce. Set aside.

Place the fish in a steamer basket. Steam over boiling water for 7 to 8 minutes, or until the fish flakes easily with a fork. Serve topped with the salsa.

Serves 4

MICRO METHOD: Fish in a Flash

Credit the microwave with being one of the fastest—and healthiest—ways to cook fish. Because the microwave speeds cooking, there's little moisture loss. That means you'll be eating tender, moist, and succulent fish that doesn't *need* a fatty sauce to taste good.

One pound of fish cooks in roughly 4 to 5 minutes. That's enough fish for four servings—at about a minute per serving. You won't find anything more convenient than that! Here are some tips for getting the best results.

■ Small items, such as shrimp and bay scallops, cook more quickly than whole fish and thick steaks.

■ Always peel shrimp before microwaving. Microwaving can make the shells difficult to remove.

■ To prevent overcooking, choose fish fillets of uniform thickness. If the fillets are irregular, overlap thinner pieces to build them up. Or fold the thinner parts under.

■ Cook fish directly on a plate or in a casserole dish. Do not use paper towels, as the fish may stick.

■ Rotate the dish or rearrange the fish after half the cooking time.

■ Cover the dish to facilitate cooking. Pour off any excess liquid that accumulates before serving.

■ Remove fish from the oven when it's barely cooked. Let stand, covered, for a few minutes, then test for doneness. The flesh should be opaque and easy to flake with a fork.

■ If your recipe contains longer-cooking ingredients, such as carrots or

(continued)

FISH—*CONTINUED*

potatoes, partially cook them first. Add the seafood toward the end.

■ Remember that fish will begin cooking as soon as it is combined with hot foods or sauces. To avoid overcooking, you may want to reduce power to medium (50 percent).

■ If using full power, stir casseroles often and check fillets and steaks frequently to avoid overcooking. Remove shellfish cooked on high power from the oven while still translucent and allow them to stand for a few minutes to finish cooking.

■ For best results, defrost frozen fish in the refrigerator. Just place it on a plate in the fridge in the morning if you intend serving it for dinner. If you defrost the fish in the microwave and then cook it there, too, you may find the flavor and texture unpleasantly changed. Also, since fish cooks so rapidly, it's difficult to defrost it without actually cooking the flesh.

■ For nice flavor, you may want to add a small amount of herbs (fresh if possible), spices, flavored vinegar, lemon juice, or lime juice before cooking. Or cook the fish on a bed of shredded vegetables.

■ To cook several fillets, you might want to use this pinwheel method: Fold under the *thick* end of the fillets and arrange them facing toward the outside of a shallow dish. Position the thinner ends pointing toward the center of the dish. Microwaves tend to cook foods from the circumference of the dish toward the center, so this arrangement ensures even cooking.

■ Similarly, arrange fish steaks pinwheel fashion, with the wide ends toward the outside of the dish.

■ When cooking whole fish, you have the option of removing the head and tail or leaving them on. For added flavor, place some chopped vegetables or herbs inside the cavity.

■ When cooking fillets in sauce, reduce the amount of liquid in the sauce, since there will be no evaporation during the short cooking time. Because sauce will shield delicate fish, there is no need to cover the dish. Besides, excess steam produced by covering might make the sauce watery.

OYSTER STEW

◇ *Per serving*

*179 calories
3.2 g. fat
(16% of calories)
2.5 g. dietary fiber
48 mg. cholesterol
202 mg. sodium*

1 pint oysters with liquid (about 2 dozen)
3 tablespoons water
1 cup minced onions
1 cup minced mushrooms
½ cup minced celery

2 cups defatted chicken stock
1½ cups diced potatoes
¼ cup minced fresh parsley
1 bay leaf
½ teaspoon dried thyme

1½ cups skim milk
1 tablespoon lemon juice
¼ teaspoon paprika
¼ cup julienned scallions

*R*emove the oysters from their liquid. Strain the liquid through a cheesecloth-lined sieve and reserve.

Rinse the oysters, rubbing lightly to loosen grit and sand. Place in a strainer to drain.

In a 4-quart pot, bring the water to a boil. Add the onions, mushrooms, and celery. Cover the pan and steam the vegetables over low heat for 5 minutes, stirring occasionally.

Add the stock, potatoes, parsley, bay leaf, and thyme. Bring to a boil. Reduce the heat, cover, and simmer for 10 minutes, or until the potatoes are tender.

Add the oysters, reserved liquid, milk, lemon juice, and paprika. Heat gently for about 5 minutes (do not let boil). Discard the bay leaf. Sprinkle with the scallions.

Serves 4

CHAPTER TEN ◇

Perfect Poultry and Game

Poultry is probably the most versatile meat in the world. It takes nicely to the flavors of other ingredients and lends itself to all manner of low-fat cooking methods. And game is now being recognized for the lean meat it is. Together, they're an indispensable part of the low-fat kitchen.

Skinless turkey breast is the undisputed king of the roost. It's about as low in fat as a meat can get, and you don't need to roast a whole bird to enjoy its benefits. Boneless, skinless cutlets are readily available and tailor-made for healthy cooking. That's why we're featuring so many delicious ways to enjoy this cut. Take your choice of Honey-Basil Turkey, Moroccan Turkey, Sautéed Turkey with Strawberry Puree, Turkey Cutlets with Pear-Pecan Stuffing, and more.

For variety, turn to boneless chicken breast. It's just marginally higher in fat than turkey but every bit as desirable from a health, taste, and convenience standpoint. It's superb for all types of international dishes, including Chinese Chicken, Curried Chicken Breasts, and Jamaican Chicken.

If you crave a different taste sensation or just want a change of pace, give game a try. It's low in fat and increasingly available in local markets. Rabbit, venison, and buffalo, for example, are wonderful when seasoned with pungent herbs and spices. Dishes such as Chinese-Style Rabbit, Venison Brochettes, and Buffalo Chili are no-fuss introductions to these new foods.

APRICOT-STUFFED HENS

◇ *Per serving*

588 calories
12.5 g. fat
(19% of calories)
4.4 g. dietary fiber
0 mg. cholesterol
293 mg. sodium

1 cup apple
juice
1 cup apricot
nectar
2 teaspoons
low-sodium
soy sauce
½ teaspoon
crushed
cardamom

½ teaspoon
ground
ginger
¼ teaspoon
black pepper
4 Cornish hens
1½ cups defatted
stock
½ cup wild rice

1 bay leaf
1 cup minced
onions
1 cup chopped
dried
apricots
2 tablespoons
pine nuts

*I*n a 9 × 13-inch baking dish, combine the apple juice, apricot nectar, soy sauce, cardamom, ginger, and pepper. Add the hens and turn to coat. Allow to marinate for 30 to 60 minutes.

In a 1-quart saucepan, combine the stock, wild rice, and bay leaf. Bring to a boil. Cover, reduce the heat, and simmer for 40 minutes, or until the rice is tender and the liquid has been absorbed. Discard the bay leaf.

Remove the hens from the marinade (reserve the marinade).

In a 2-quart saucepan, cook the onions in 2 tablespoons of the marinade until wilted, about 5 minutes. Add the apricots, pine nuts, and rice. Heat through, adding more marinade if the mixture is too dry.

Distribute the stuffing among the hens, filling the cavities. (Place any remaining stuffing in a small casserole dish that you've coated with nonstick spray.)

Coat a roasting pan with nonstick spray. Add the hens. Bake at 350°F for 45 minutes, basting occasionally with the marinade. Add the casserole dish to the oven and bake for 15 minutes more, or until the hens are tender when pierced with a fork. If the hens appear to be getting too brown, cover with foil.

Transfer the remaining marinade to a 1-quart saucepan. Boil until reduced by half. Serve as a sauce with the hens. Remove the skin before eating.

Serves 4

Turkey Cutlets with Pear-Pecan Stuffing

◇ *Per serving*

256 calories
7.2 g. fat
(25% of calories)
2.9 g. dietary fiber
68 mg. cholesterol
151 mg. sodium

½ cup minced celery
¼ cup minced shallots
½ cup defatted chicken stock
¼ cup chopped pecans
1 cup diced pears

½ cup whole wheat bread crumbs
¾ teaspoon dried thyme
⅛ teaspoon ground allspice
1 pound turkey cutlets

¼ cup pear juice
2 tablespoons snipped chives
2 tablespoons minced fresh parsley

*I*n a large nonstick frying pan, sauté the celery and shallots in ¼ cup of the stock until soft, about 4 minutes. Stir in the pecans and toast for 1 minute. Remove from the heat.

Add the pears, bread crumbs, thyme, allspice, and 1 tablespoon of the remaining stock.

Place the cutlets between sheets of waxed paper or plastic wrap and pound to an even thickness (about ⅓ to ½ inch) with a mallet.

Divide the stuffing among the cutlets, mounding it in the center of each. Carefully roll up each cutlet to enclose stuffing (if necessary tie with a string or use skewers).

Coat a 9 × 9-inch baking dish with nonstick spray. Add the cutlets. Lightly mist the top of each with nonstick spray.

In a cup, combine the remaining 3 tablespoons stock and the pear juice. Spoon over the cutlets. Cover the dish tightly with foil.

Bake at 350°F for 20 minutes. Remove the foil. Bake, basting occasionally, for 10 to 15 minutes, or until lightly browned.

Sprinkle with the chives and parsley.

Serves 4

MICRO METHOD: Bird Talk

There are several reasons to reach for the microwave when cooking poultry. One is the expected savings of time. Most poultry microwaved on full power is table-ready in one-third to one-half the time that conventional methods require. (Stewing hens are an exception. Because they are large and best microwaved at 50 percent power, they take nearly as long as conventional cooking. Further, the skin will not become tender. You're better off using another method.)

Another advantage to microwaving most birds is that dark meat is less likely to discolor next to the bone. Also, white meat remains nice and moist. But the most important health advantage is that microwaving does a good job of liquefying fat so it drains off. For best drainage, cook poultry on a microwave drainer or ridged microwave rack. If you'd like to brown the meat, microwave it until almost done, then grill or broil as desired.

Because microwaves cook food from the circumference of a dish toward the center, always position the parts of chicken that take longest to cook—the dark meat and thick sections of white meat—toward the outside of your dish. When cooking a split chicken breast, arrange it so that the thick breastbone sections face outward. If doing several split breasts, arrange them pinwheel fashion, with the thin pointed ends toward the center and the meatier sections toward the outside.

Cooking a small amount of chicken for salad is simple in the microwave. Allow one-half boneless, skinless breast per person and cook it on full power just until opaque. Four breast halves cook in as little as 5 minutes in a full-size microwave; smaller quantities take less time.

When using poultry in a casserole, reduce the liquid by one-third to one-half (unless the liquid is needed to rehydrate dry pasta or rice). Because brown rice requires longer cooking than most poultry, cook the rice by itself until almost tender, then add the chicken.

STEAMED WONTONS

◇ *Per serving*

106 calories
1.1 g. fat
(9% of calories)
0.1 g. dietary fiber
22 mg. cholesterol
332 mg. sodium

WONTONS
8 ounces boneless, skinless chicken breasts
¼ cup minced scallions
1 teaspoon low-sodium soy sauce
1 teaspoon peeled grated gingerroot
¼ teaspoon honey
1 clove garlic, minced
24 round wonton skins

SAUCE
3 tablespoons low-sodium soy sauce
3 tablespoons defatted stock
½ teaspoon sesame oil

*T*o make the wontons: Cut the chicken into 1-inch pieces. In a food processor, combine the chicken, scallions, soy sauce, ginger, honey, and garlic with on/off turns until finely chopped.

Place 1 teaspoon of filling in the center of each wonton skin. Lightly moisten the circumference with water so edges will stick together. Pleat the edges around the filling so the wontons resemble flowers.

Steam over boiling water in batches for 8 to 10 minutes.

To make the sauce: In a small bowl, combine the soy sauce, stock, and oil. Use as a dipping sauce for the wontons.

Serves 6

◇   ◇   ◇

CHINESE CHICKEN

◇ *Per serving*

149 calories
2.7 g. fat
(16% of calories)
0.8 g. dietary fiber
66 mg. cholesterol
77 mg. sodium

1 pound boneless, skinless chicken breasts
2 cloves garlic, crushed
1 teaspoon peeled minced gingerroot
1 green pepper, julienned
4 scallions, julienned
2 tablespoons vinegar
1 teaspoon sesame oil
1 head green lettuce

*I*n a large frying pan over medium heat, combine the chicken, garlic, and ginger. Add cold water to cover. Bring to a simmer, cover, and cook until the chicken is tender, about 10 to 15 minutes. Drain the chicken and place in the refrigerator to chill.

Shred the chicken and place in a large bowl. Add the peppers and scallions.

In a small bowl, whisk together the vinegar and oil. Pour over the chicken and toss well to combine.

To serve, mound the chicken on a serving platter. Divide the head of lettuce into individual leaves. Place a little chicken on each lettuce leaf, roll, and eat.

Serves 4

◇ ◇ ◇

MARINADE MAGIC FOR POULTRY

Tasty, low-fat marinades impart great flavor to poultry. And they're excellent for basting the meat as it cooks to help keep it juicy. For best results, simply skin the poultry and place it in a large bowl or shallow baking dish with the marinade. Flip the pieces often to ensure even coverage. Cover the meat and let stand at room temperature for no longer than 1 hour. Then cook immediately. For longer marinating, place the poultry in the refrigerator.

Here are five tasty marinades suitable for any type of poultry. Vary the proportions to suit your taste.

■ Defatted chicken stock, minced garlic, minced fresh ginger, low-sodium soy sauce, and grated orange rind
■ Tomato juice, minced garlic, minced fresh oregano, ground cumin, and ground coriander
■ Buttermilk, curry powder, and minced fresh coriander or parsley
■ Defatted chicken stock, minced fresh thyme, ground black pepper, dried mustard, and ground red pepper
■ Defatted chicken stock, lemon juice, minced onions, minced garlic, minced fresh oregano, and crushed celery seeds

CURRIED CHICKEN BREASTS

¼ cup defatted chicken stock
3 cloves garlic, minced
2 teaspoons curry powder
2 teaspoons honey
1 teaspoon dried marjoram
1 teaspoon ground fennel
1 teaspoon ground cumin
1 teaspoon ground coriander
½ teaspoon ground fenugreek
½ teaspoon red pepper flakes
½ teaspoon saffron
⅛ teaspoon black pepper
½ cup nonfat yogurt
1 pound boneless, skinless chicken breasts

*I*n a large nonstick frying pan over medium-high heat, combine the stock, garlic, curry powder, honey, marjoram, fennel, cumin, coriander, fenugreek, pepper-flakes, saffron, and black pepper. Simmer, stirring constantly, until the spices are fragrant, about 3 minutes. Remove from the heat and let cool for 5 minutes. Whisk in the yogurt.

Place the chicken breasts between sheets of waxed paper or plastic wrap and pound to an even thickness (about ⅓ to ½ inch) with a mallet. Place the chicken in the spice mixture and turn to coat. Marinate for about 30 minutes, flipping the pieces occasionally.

Coat a 9 × 13-inch baking dish with nonstick spray. Add the chicken. Bake at 350°F until cooked through, about 20 minutes.

Serves 4

◇ ◇ ◇

DIAMOND HEAD TURKEY WITH PINEAPPLE

◇ **Per serving**

205 calories
2 g. fat
(9% of calories)
2.4 g. dietary fiber
51 mg. cholesterol
358 mg. sodium

12 ounces turkey cutlets
½ cup pineapple juice
½ cup minced onions
3 tablespoons apple-cider vinegar
2 tablespoons low-sodium soy sauce

1 tablespoon peeled minced gingerroot
3 cloves garlic, minced
1 ripe pineapple
1 tablespoon cornstarch

1 green pepper, cut into thin strips
1 sweet red pepper, cut into thin strips

Cut the turkey into bite-size pieces.

In a large bowl, combine the pineapple juice, onions, vinegar, soy sauce, ginger, and garlic. Add the turkey. Cover and refrigerate for 4 hours.

Peel, core, and slice the pineapple into ½-inch cubes.

Drain the turkey and onions, reserving the marinade.

Heat a large nonstick frying pan over medium-high heat. Add 3 tablespoons of the marinade and heat for 1 minute. Add the turkey and onions. Stir-fry just until brown. Remove from the pan and keep warm.

Dissolve the cornstarch in the remaining marinade. Add to the pan. Cook, stirring constantly, until thick.

Add the green peppers, red peppers, pineapple, and turkey mixture. Toss to coat with sauce and reheat the turkey.

Serves 4

Turkey and Shrimp Kabobs with Tomatoes

◇ *Per serving*

330 calories
6 g. fat
(16% of calories)
3.7 g. dietary fiber
111 mg. cholesterol
136 mg. sodium

8 ounces boneless, skinless turkey breast
8 ounces shrimp, peeled and deveined
2 tablespoons lemon juice
¼ cup minced fresh parsley
4 cloves garlic, minced

1 jalapeño pepper, minced
2 tablespoons minced shallots
1 tablespoon olive oil
1 teaspoon red-pepper flakes

1 teaspoon dried basil
1½ pounds tomatoes, peeled, seeded, and chopped
2 cups hot cooked rice

Cut the turkey into 1-inch cubes. Combine in a large bowl with the shrimp and lemon juice. Cover and let stand about 30 minutes.

In a large frying pan, combine the parsley, garlic, peppers, shallots, oil, pepper flakes, and basil. Sauté over medium heat for 5 minutes. Add the tomatoes, cover the pan, and cook for 10 minutes.

Thread the turkey and shrimp onto skewers. Broil about 4 inches from the heat until cooked through, about 3 minutes per side.

Serve with the rice and cooked tomatoes.

Serves 4

Rabbit Sauté
with Mushrooms

◇ *Per serving*

504 calories
13.5 g. fat
(24% of calories)
2.9 g. dietary fiber
65 mg. cholesterol
123 mg. sodium

2 pounds rabbit pieces
4 tablespoons flour
2 teaspoons olive oil
2¼ cups defatted chicken stock
2 cups sliced shiitake mushrooms
1 large onion, sliced crosswise into rings
2 tablespoons vinegar
2 cloves garlic, minced
1 teaspoon Dijon mustard
½ teaspoon dried thyme
1 bay leaf
8 ounces broad noodles
½ cup minced fresh parsley

Dredge the rabbit in the flour.

In a large nonstick frying pan over medium heat, sauté the rabbit in the oil until golden, about 5 minutes on each side.

Add the stock, mushrooms, onions, vinegar, garlic, mustard, thyme, and bay leaf. Stir to combine. Bring to a boil. Lower the heat and cover loosely. Simmer until tender, about 40 minutes, stirring occasionally.

Cook the noodles in a large pot of boiling water until tender. Drain and transfer to a serving platter. Add the rabbit and sauce. Sprinkle with the parsley.

Serves 4

VENISON BROCHETTES

4 cloves garlic, minced
2 teaspoons orange juice
½ teaspoon grated orange rind
½ teaspoon ground mace
½ teaspoon ground cumin
⅛ teaspoon ground cinnamon
⅛ teaspoon ground ginger
½ cup nonfat yogurt
1 pound venison saddle or loin
2 cups hot cooked rice

*I*n a large bowl, combine the garlic, orange juice, orange rind, mace, cumin, cinnamon, and ginger. Whisk in the yogurt.

Cut the venison into 1½-inch cubes. Add to the yogurt mixture and stir to combine well. Cover and refrigerate overnight. Stir occasionally.

Thread the venison onto skewers, taking care not to crowd the pieces. Reserve the yogurt. Broil about 5 inches from the heat, turning frequently and basting with leftover yogurt mixture, until cooked through, about 10 to 12 minutes.

Serve over the rice.

Serves 4

◇ ◇

MOROCCAN TURKEY

1 pound turkey cutlets
2 teaspoons olive oil
½ teaspoon ground ginger
½ teaspoon ground cinnamon
¼ teaspoon ground cumin
⅛ teaspoon ground red pepper
⅛ teaspoon turmeric
1 tablespoon ground almonds
2 tablespoons honey

*P*lace the cutlets between sheets of waxed paper or plastic wrap and pound to an even thickness (about 1/3 to 1/2 inch) with a mallet.

In a pie plate, combine the oil, ginger, cinnamon, cumin, red pepper, and turmeric. Dip the turkey in the mixture to coat both sides of each cutlet.

Place in a large nonstick frying pan in a single layer. Sprinkle with the almonds and drizzle with the honey.

Cover the pan and cook over medium-high heat for 8 to 10 minutes, or until the turkey is opaque. Do not overcook.

Serves 4

◇   ◇   ◇

CHINESE-STYLE RABBIT

◇ *Per serving*

522 calories
13.7 g. fat
(24% of calories)
2.5 g. dietary fiber
65 mg. cholesterol
245 mg. sodium

1 tablespoon canola oil	1 tablespoon honey	1 teaspoon hot-pepper sauce
2 pounds rabbit pieces	1 teaspoon peeled minced gingerroot	4 cups hot cooked rice
1½ cups defatted chicken stock	4 cloves garlic, minced	
2 tablespoons tomato paste		
1 tablespoon low-sodium soy sauce		

*I*n a large nonstick frying pan over medium heat, heat the oil. Add the rabbit and sauté until it begins to brown, about 5 minutes.

In a medium bowl, combine the stock, tomato paste, soy sauce, honey, ginger, garlic, and hot-pepper sauce. Pour over the rabbit.

Reduce the heat to medium-low, partially cover the pan, and simmer the rabbit until cooked through, about 20 to 25 minutes.

Serve with the rice.

Serves 4

GRILLED CHICKEN AND ARTICHOKES WITH MIXED GREENS

◇ *Per serving*

263 calories
7 g. fat
(24% of calories)
1.6 g. dietary fiber
66 mg. cholesterol
167 mg. sodium

2 bunches arugula
1 head radicchio
3 ounces alfalfa sprouts
12 artichoke hearts, halved
8 sun-dried tomatoes, sliced, or cherry tomatoes, halved

1 sweet yellow pepper, thinly sliced
1 pound boneless, skinless chicken breasts
⅓ cup balsamic vinegar

1½ tablespoons olive oil
1 tablespoon minced fresh basil or thyme
¼ teaspoon ground black pepper

Divide the arugula, radicchio, sprouts, artichokes, tomatoes, and peppers among serving plates. Set aside.

Grill or broil the chicken for about 5 minutes per side, or until cooked through. Slice as desired and place on the greens.

In a small bowl, whisk together the vinegar, oil, basil or thyme, and pepper. Spoon over the salad.

Serves 4

Ginger Turkey
with Spicy Tomato Sauce

12 ounces turkey cutlets
1¼ cups nonfat yogurt
¼ cup tomato puree
1 tablespoon paprika
2 teaspoons turmeric
2 cloves garlic, minced
1 tablespoon peeled grated gingerroot
1 teaspoon ground cinnamon
1 teaspoon ground cardamom
¼ teaspoon ground cloves
¼ teaspoon red pepper
2 teaspoons canola oil
1 sweet red pepper, cut into ¼-inch strips

Cut the turkey into 1-inch strips. Place in a large bowl and add ½ cup yogurt. Combine well, cover, and marinate in the refrigerator for 2 to 3 hours.

In a small bowl, whisk together the remaining yogurt, tomato puree, paprika, and turmeric. Set aside.

In another small bowl, combine the garlic, ginger, cinnamon, cardamom, cloves, and red pepper. Set aside.

Drain the turkey of excess marinade and pat dry with paper towels.

In a large nonstick frying pan over medium-high heat, heat the oil. Add the turkey and brown on all sides. Remove from the pan.

Add the spice mixture to the pan and cook over low heat, stirring constantly, until fragrant, about 1 minutes. Then immediately add the yogurt mixture to the pan. Bring to a boil.

Return the turkey to the pan. Add the red peppers. Simmer for 10 minutes, or until the sauce thickens and coats the turkey.

Serves 4

Honey-Basil Turkey

◇ *Per serving*

177 calories
2.1 g. fat
(11% of calories)
<0.1 g. dietary fiber
68 mg. cholesterol
349 mg. sodium

½ cup apple-cider vinegar
¼ cup minced fresh basil
2 tablespoons Dijon mustard
2 tablespoons honey

1 tablespoon low-sodium soy sauce
3 cloves garlic, minced

½ teaspoon dried thyme
1 pound turkey cutlets

*I*n a shallow baking dish, combine the vinegar, basil, mustard, honey, soy sauce, garlic, and thyme.

Add the turkey and turn to coat. Cover and marinate for 15 minutes.

Remove the turkey from the marinade. Transfer the marinade to a large frying pan. Place the turkey on a broiler rack. Broil about 6 inches from the heat until cooked through, about 5 minutes per side.

Bring the marinade to a boil and cook until reduced by half, about 5 minutes. Add the turkey and reheat briefly.

Serves 4

Summer Chicken Salad Sandwiches

◇ *Per serving*

335 calories
6.9 g. fat
(19% of calories)
5.1 g. dietary fiber
54 mg. cholesterol
471 mg. sodium

3 cups cubed cooked chicken breast
½ cup halved grapes
¼ cup minced scallions
¼ cup minced fresh parsley

2 tablespoons chopped pecans
½ cup nonfat yogurt
2 tablespoons nonfat mayonnaise

1½ teaspoons curry powder
12 slices pumpernickel bread
2 nectarines, thinly sliced

*I*n a large bowl, combine the chicken, grapes, scallions, parsley, and pecans.

In a cup, combine the yogurt, mayonnaise, and curry powder. Mix the dressing with the chicken.

Divide the chicken among six slices of the bread. Top with the nectarines and the remaining bread.

Serves 6

◇   ◇   ◇

SAUTÉED TURKEY WITH STRAWBERRY PUREE

◇ *Per serving*

208 calories
5.5 g. fat
(24% of calories)
2.4 g. dietary fiber
68 mg. cholesterol
72 mg. sodium

1 pound turkey cutlets	1 tablespoon canola oil	1 teaspoon honey
¼ cup whole wheat flour	1½ cups sliced strawberries	

*P*lace the cutlets between sheets of waxed paper or plastic wrap and pound to an even thickness (about ⅓ to ½ inch) with a mallet. Lightly dredge the cutlets in the flour; shake off the excess.

In a large nonstick frying pan over medium-high heat, sauté the turkey in the oil for 3 minutes per side, or until cooked through. Remove to a platter and keep warm.

In a blender or food processor, puree half of the strawberries. Add to the frying pan with the honey and stir until heated. Add the remaining strawberries and fold in gently.

Spoon the sauce over the turkey.

Serves 4

JAMAICAN CHICKEN

◇ *Per serving*

125 calories
1.3 g. fat
(9% of calories)
0.4 g. dietary fiber
49 mg. cholesterol
226 mg. sodium

⅓ cup defatted chicken stock
1 tablespoon low-sodium soy sauce
1 teaspoon peeled minced gingerroot
1 bay leaf
1 clove garlic, minced

¼ teaspoon ground allspice
12 ounces boneless, skinless chicken breasts
½ cup sliced mushrooms

½ cup thinly sliced yellow peppers
½ cup sliced celery
1 teaspoon cornstarch
1 teaspoon honey

*I*n a large bowl, combine the stock, soy sauce, ginger, bay leaf, garlic, and allspice.

Cut the chicken into ¼-inch strips. Add to the bowl and stir well. Cover, refrigerate, and marinate for at least 4 hours, stirring occasionally. Remove the chicken from the bowl and reserve the marinade. Discard the bay leaf.

Coat a large nonstick frying pan with nonstick spray. Stir-fry the chicken over medium-high heat for 3 to 5 minutes, adding a bit of marinade if necessary to prevent scorching. Remove the chicken and drain on paper towels. Transfer to a bowl. Wipe the pan clean.

In the same pan over medium-high heat, sauté the mushrooms, peppers, and celery with 1 tablespoon of the marinade for 1 minute. Add the vegetables to the chicken.

In a small bowl, combine the remaining marinade with the cornstarch and honey.

Pour into the frying pan and heat, stirring constantly, until thick and shiny. Add the chicken and vegetables. Toss to coat with sauce.

Serves 4

perfect poultry and game

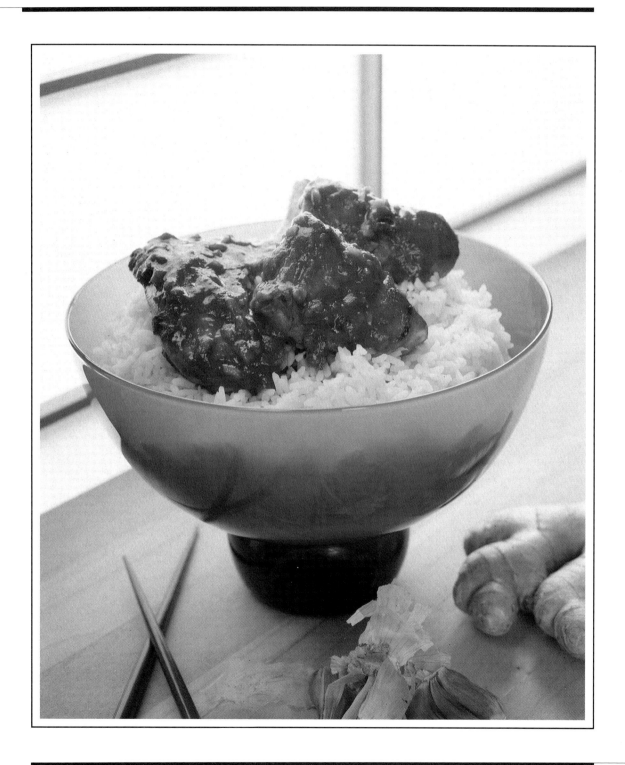

CHINESE-STYLE RABBIT (PAGE 227)

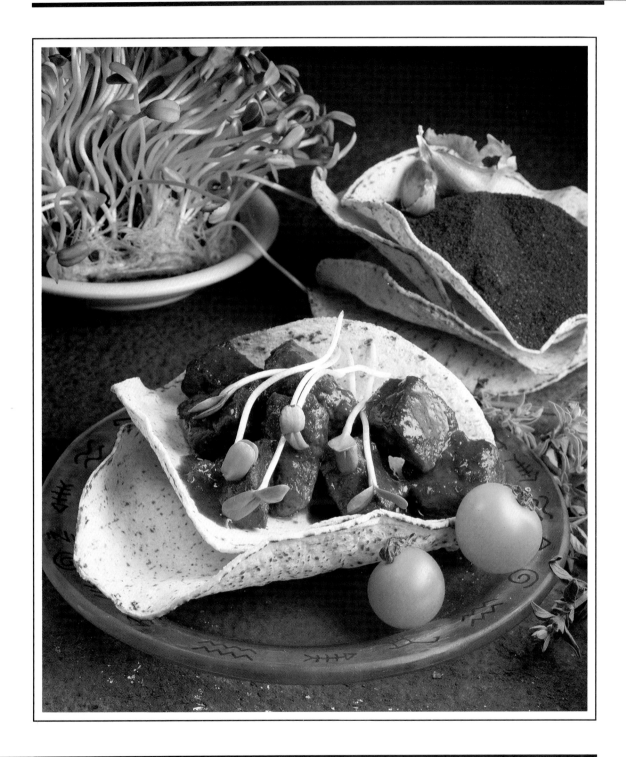

Buffalo Chili (page 250)

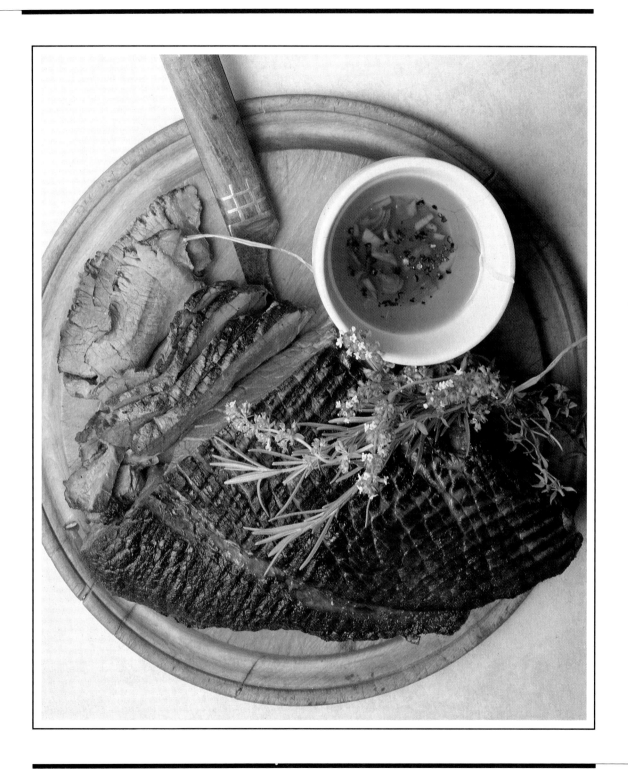

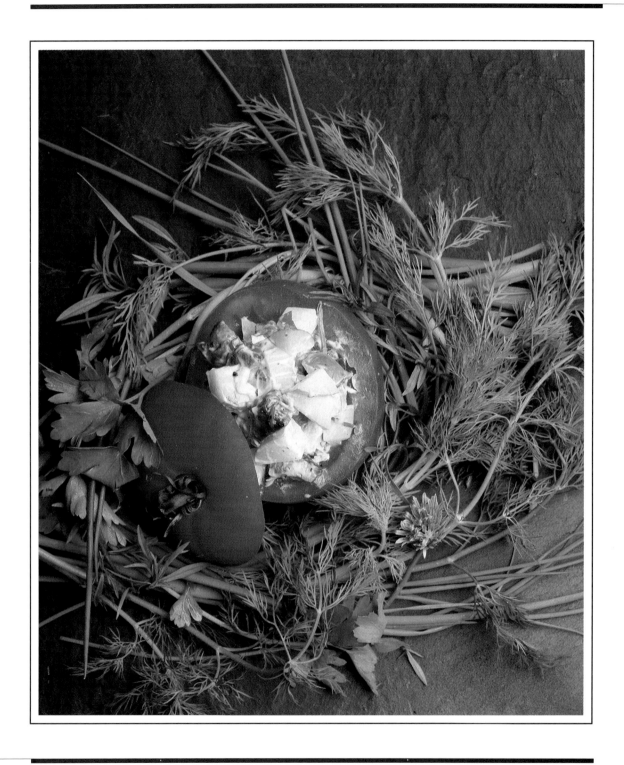

Tomatoes Stuffed with Lamb Hash (page 258)

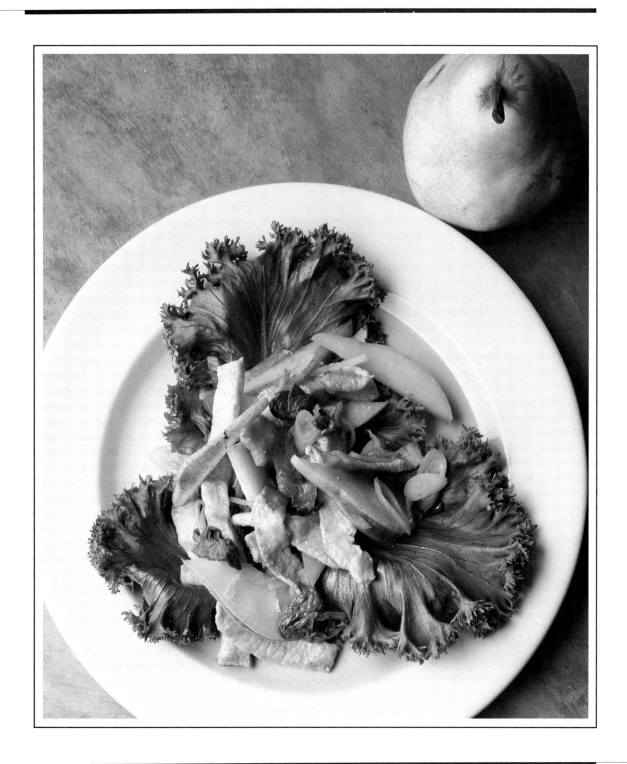

PEAR AND PORK STIR-FRY (PAGE 268)

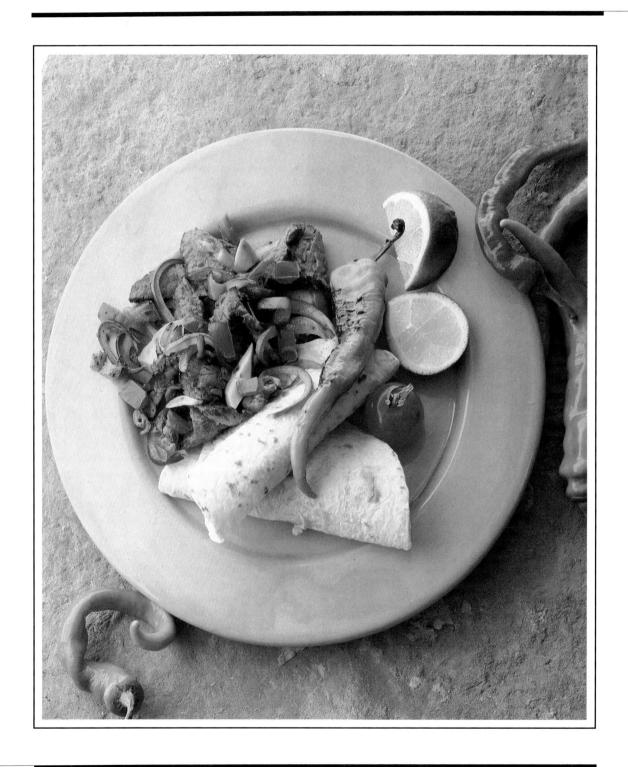

Sizzling Fajitas (page 260)

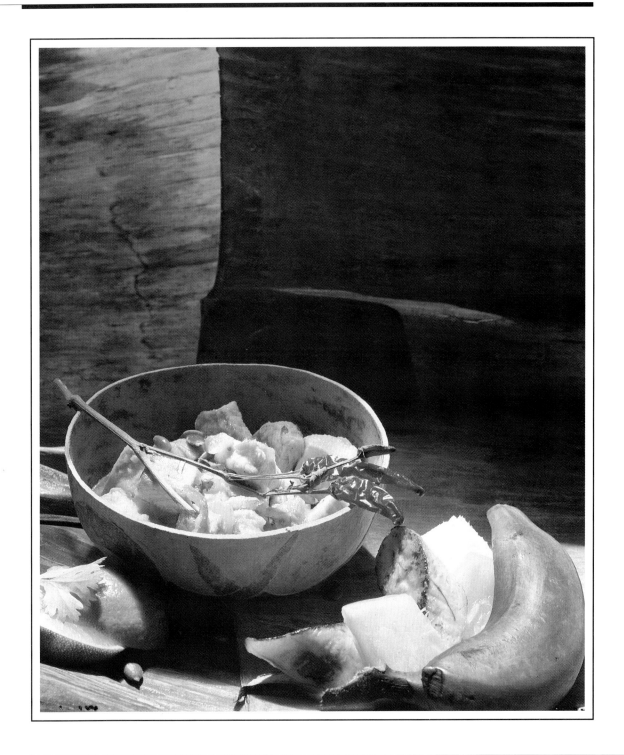

SPICY PORK AND CHICKEN WITH PINEAPPLE (PAGE 255)   239

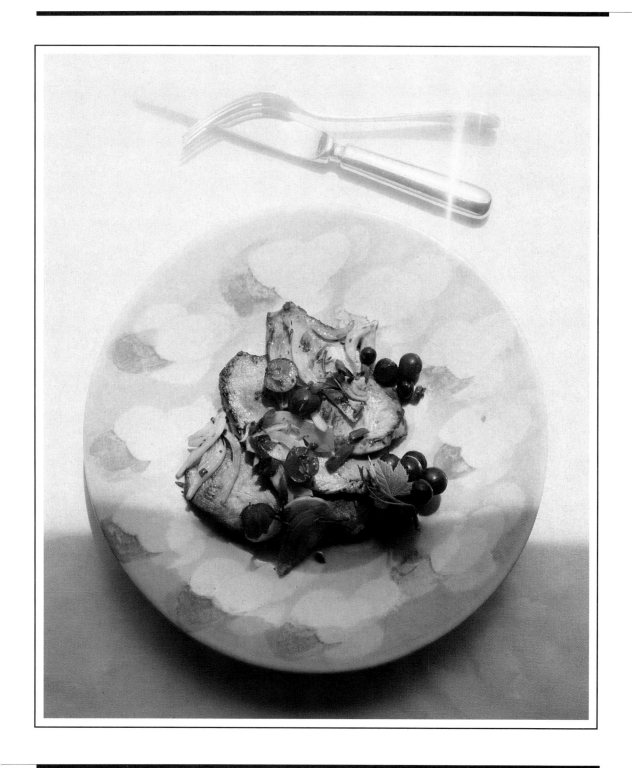

SCALLOPS OF VEAL WITH FENNEL AND GRAPES (PAGE 265)

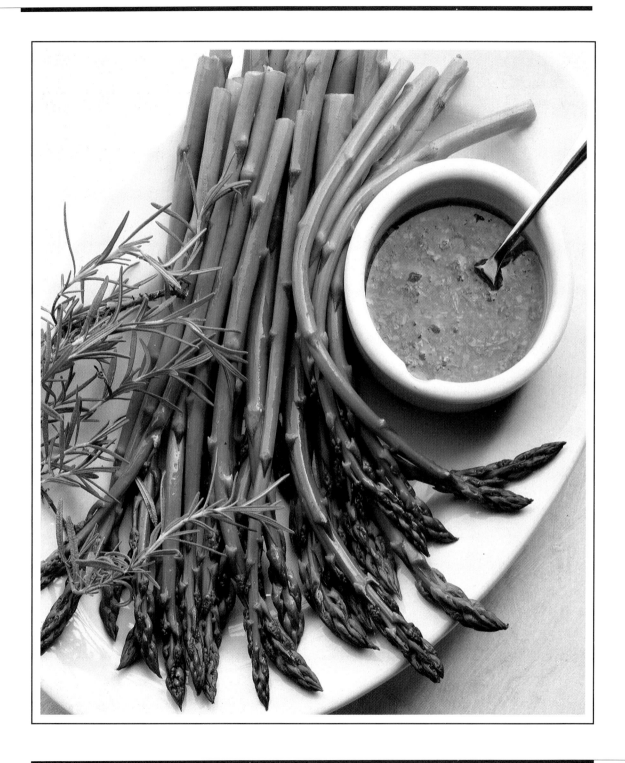

ROSEMARY ASPARAGUS (PAGE 284)

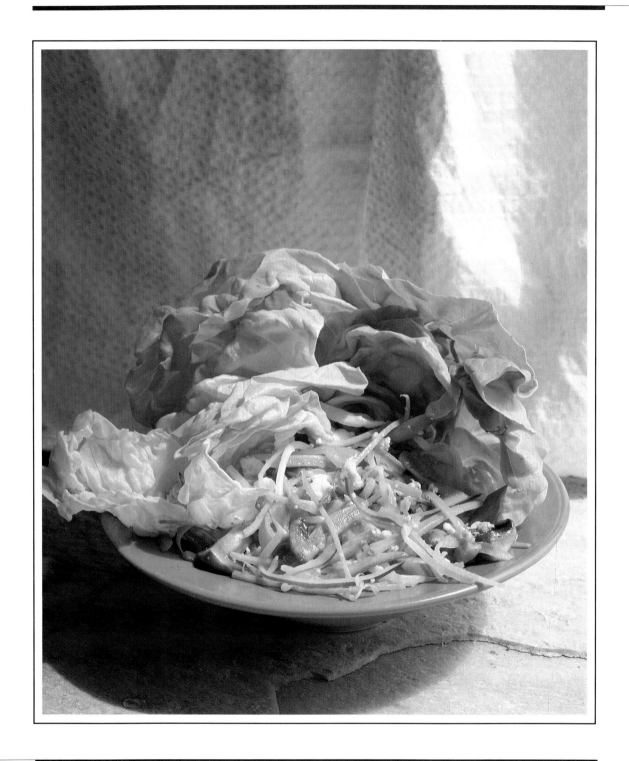

VEGETABLE EGG ROLL-UPS (PAGE 286)

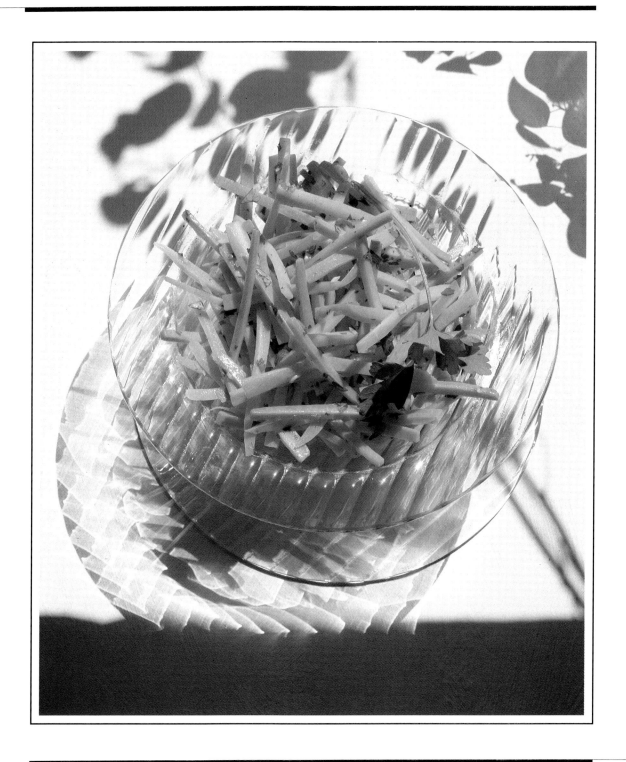

MOROCCAN CARROT SALAD (PAGE 280)

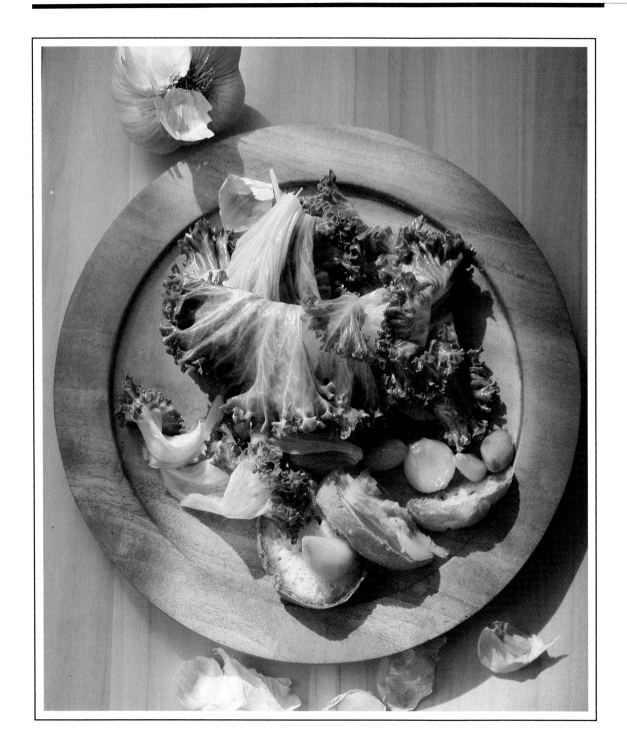

GREENS WITH GARLIC (PAGE 276)

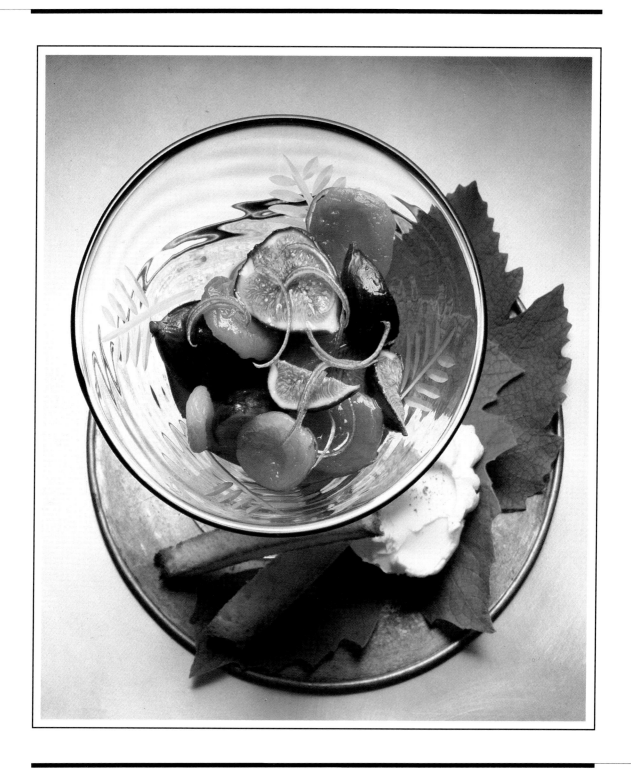

MARINATED FIGS AND APRICOTS (PAGE 294)

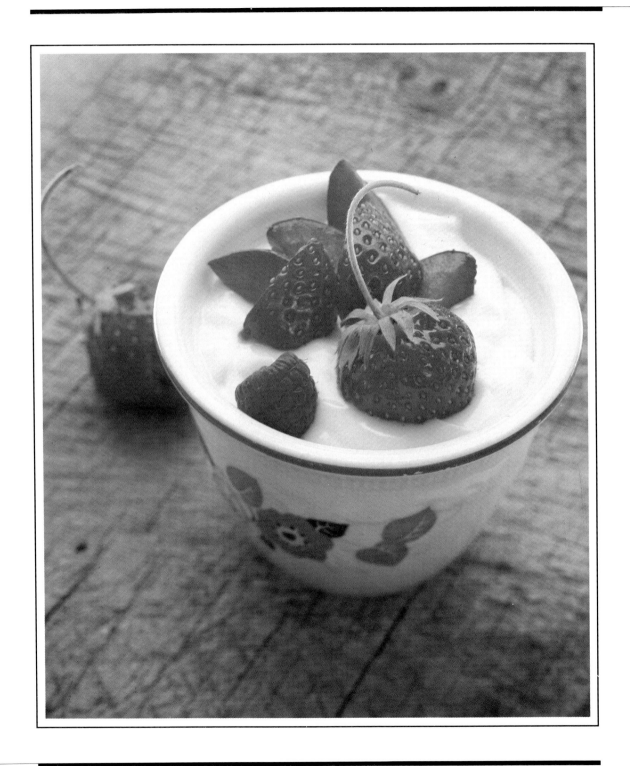

BERRY CUSTARD (PAGE 299)

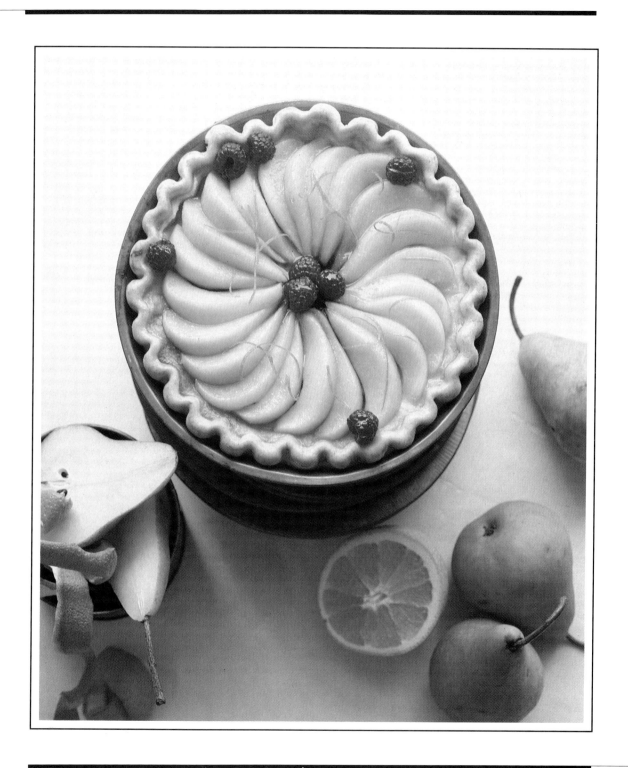

PEAR-CHEESE PIE (PAGE 289)

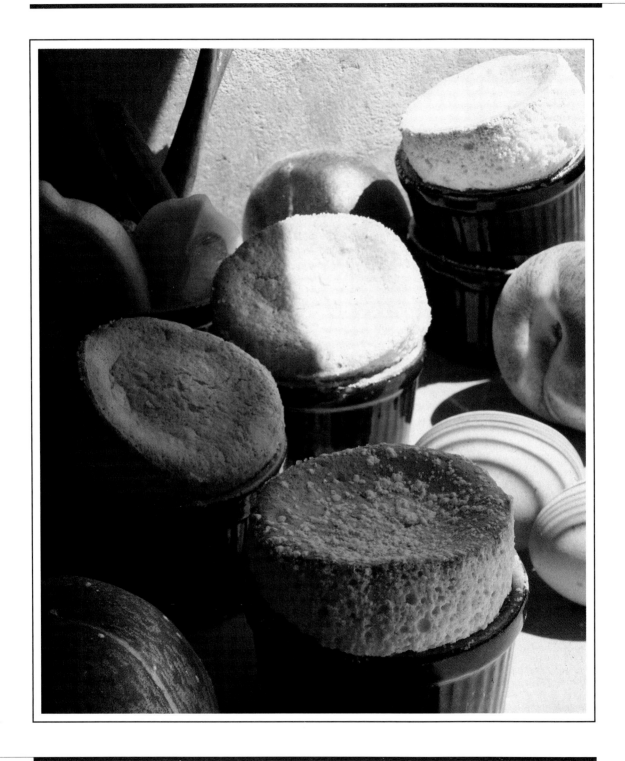

PEACH SOUFFLÉ (PAGE 294)

CHICKEN
WITH TROPICAL FRUIT

◇ *Per serving*

251 calories
5.4 g. fat
(19% of calories)
1.9 g. dietary fiber
67 mg. cholesterol
126 mg. sodium

1 papaya, thinly sliced
1 star fruit, sliced
1 banana, sliced
1 tablespoon lime juice
1 pound boneless, skinless chicken breasts
1 tablespoon olive oil
¼ cup defatted chicken stock
2 teaspoons curry powder
1 cup nonfat yogurt

*I*n a large bowl, combine the papayas, star fruit, bananas, and lime juice.

Place the chicken breasts between sheets of waxed paper or plastic wrap and pound to an even thickness (about ⅓ to ½ inch) with a mallet.

Heat a large, heavy cast-iron frying pan on high for 3 minutes. Add half of the oil and half of the chicken. Sauté for 5 minutes per side. Transfer to the bowl with the fruit and toss to combine.

Repeat with the remaining oil and chicken.

Using the same frying pan, heat the stock until just boiling. Scrape the bottom with a wooden spoon to incorporate any browned bits. Add the curry powder and stir to form a paste. Transfer to a small bowl. Stir in the yogurt.

Arrange the chicken and fruit on a serving platter. Drizzle with the yogurt.

Serves 4

BUFFALO CHILI

◇ *Per serving*

343 calories
9.1 g. fat
(24% of calories)
4.9 g. dietary fiber
70 mg. cholesterol
219 mg. sodium

1 pound buffalo top round
2 tablespoons whole wheat flour
½ teaspoon dried oregano
½ teaspoon ground coriander
½ teaspoon ground cumin
⅛ teaspoon ground allspice
1 tablespoon olive oil
1⅔ cups defatted beef stock
2 tablespoons chili powder
3 cloves garlic, minced
½ teaspoon hot-pepper sauce
1 bay leaf
8 corn tortillas, warmed

Cut the buffalo into 1-inch cubes.

In a pie plate, combine the flour, oregano, coriander, cumin, and allspice. Add the meat and toss well to coat.

In a large nonstick frying pan, sauté the meat in the oil until the pieces are almost all brown.

Add the stock, chili powder, garlic, hot-pepper sauce, and bay leaf. Bring to a boil. Reduce the heat and simmer for 30 minutes, or until the meat is tender. If necessary, add more stock to prevent sticking. Discard the bay leaf.

Divide the mixture among the tortillas and roll up.

Serves 4

TURKEY CACCIATORE

8 ounces turkey cutlets
1 tablespoon whole wheat flour
2 teaspoons olive oil
¾ cup defatted chicken stock
1 large onion, thinly sliced
1 green pepper, thinly sliced
3 cloves garlic, minced
3½ cups sliced tomatoes
¾ cup thinly sliced mushrooms
¼ cup minced fresh parsley
1 teaspoon dried rosemary
½ teaspoon dried marjoram
1 bay leaf

Cut the turkey into ½-inch strips. Toss with the flour.

In a large nonstick frying pan over medium-high heat, sauté the turkey in the oil until opaque. Remove with a slotted spoon.

Add the stock to the pan and boil rapidly, scraping the bottom of the pan, until the stock is reduced by half. Reduce the heat to low and add the onion, peppers, and garlic. Cook until the vegetables are tender, about 5 minutes.

Add the tomatoes, mushrooms, parsley, rosemary, marjoram, and bay leaf. Cover and simmer 8 to 10 minutes, stirring occasionally.

Add the turkey and heat through. Discard the bay leaf.

Serves 4

ORANGE-SCENTED CHICKEN BREASTS

◇ *Per serving*

171 calories
4.2 g. fat
(22% of calories)
0.2 g. dietary fiber
66 mg. cholesterol
76 mg. sodium

2 tablespoons paprika
1 teaspoon dried oregano
½ teaspoon ground cumin
3 cloves garlic, minced

⅓ cup orange juice
3 tablespoons lime juice
2 tablespoons red-wine vinegar

2 teaspoons olive oil
1 pound boneless, skinless chicken breasts

*I*n a 9 × 13-inch baking dish, combine the paprika, oregano, cumin, and garlic. Whisk in the orange juice, lime juice, vinegar, and oil.

Place the chicken breasts between sheets of waxed paper or plastic wrap and pound to an even thickness (about ⅓ to ½ inch) with a mallet.

Add the chicken to the dish and turn to coat well. Arrange in a single layer.

Bake at 400°F, basting occasionally, for 20 minutes, or until cooked through.

Serves 4

◇ ◇ ◇

TURKEY MEDALLIONS WITH PEACHES

good
Rosemary rather Sherry

Nov 2001

◇ *Per serving*

253 calories
6.4 g. fat
(23% of calories)
3.1 g. dietary fiber

1 pound turkey cutlets
¼ cup whole wheat flour
2 teaspoons ground dried rosemary

2 cups sliced peaches
¼ cup peach nectar
¼ cup defatted chicken stock

¾ cup water
¼ cup almonds

68 mg. cholesterol
80 mg. sodium

*P*lace the cutlets between sheets of waxed paper or plastic wrap and pound to an even thickness (about ⅓ to ½ inch) with a mallet.

Combine the flour and rosemary in a pie plate. Lightly dredge the turkey in the flour; shake off the excess.

In a large nonstick frying pan over medium-high heat, cook the peaches in the nectar for about 3 minutes. Remove from the pan and reserve.

Add the stock and cutlets. Cook over medium-high heat for 1 minute on each side. Remove the pan from the heat.

In a blender, combine the water and almonds. Process on low speed until finely chopped. Pour the mixture into the pan with the turkey. Add the peaches. Return the pan to the heat and cook over low heat for 10 minutes.

Serves 4

IS IT DONE?

For maximum flavor, as well as safety, always cook poultry until well done. Here are some fail-safe ways to test a bird.

- Press the thick muscle of the drumstick. If the meat feels soft, the poultry is done.
- If cooking a whole or half bird, the leg should move up and down easily (the hip joint may even break).
- Insert a fork into the breast or a thick part of the thigh. When the meat is done, the fork slides in easily.
- Use a meat thermometer. Insert the thermometer into the fleshy inner thigh or through the carcass into the center of the stuffing. It should never touch bone. In the thigh, the thermometer should register from 180°F to 185°F when the meat is done; in the stuffing, it should read 165°F.
- Pierce the thickest part of the thigh with a skewer, a fork, or the tip of a sharp knife. The escaping juices will be clear if the meat is done.

CHAPTER ELEVEN ◇

Lean Meats

Of course you can eat meat on a healthy diet! Just choose your cuts carefully and be extra resourceful about how you prepare them. If you're unsure how to do that, let the recipes in this chapter be your guide to maximizing the health potential of red meat.

As always, start with naturally lean cuts such as flank steak, pork tenderloin, and lamb leg. And make sure to trim off every speck of visible fat. That way you get all the advantages of meat, such as lots of protein, iron, and zinc, without any of its fatty drawbacks.

That done, you can concentrate on ways to use just a little meat with a lot of other healthy ingredients. Keep portions modest (3 or 4 ounces is plenty), and combine the meat with high-fiber, nutrient-dense foods such as potatoes, pasta, beans, vegetables, grains, or even fruit. Beef recipes that follow this guideline include Orchard Meat Loaf and Mexican Picadillo. If lamb or veal is more your style, you'll like Fruited Lamb Curry or Scallops of Veal with Fennel and Grapes.

Pork, too, marries well with fruits such as pears and peaches. Pear and Pork Stir-Fry, for example, incorporates fiber-rich pears and spinach. Likewise, Peaches and Pork contains fiber plus beta-carotene to help protect against certain kinds of cancer.

For entertaining, choose impressive yet easy low-fat dishes such as London Broil with Garlic Marinade, Sizzling Fajitas, or Spicy Pork and Chicken with Pineapple. These dishes are guaranteed to please your guests and appease your good conscience. And that's one challenge worth meating!

Spicy Pork and Chicken with Pineapple

◇ *Per serving*

384 calories
9.8 g. fat
(23% of calories)
5.6 g. dietary fiber
93 mg. cholesterol
129 mg. sodium

1 pound lean pork, trimmed of all visible fat
2 tablespoons canola oil
1 onion, coarsely chopped
4 cloves garlic, halved
2½ cups defatted stock
¼ cup minced fresh coriander

3 jalapeño peppers, seeded and chopped
2 tablespoons cornmeal
1 teaspoon hot-pepper flakes
1 pound boneless, skinless chicken breasts

4 bananas
½ cup toasted pumpkin seeds
1 pineapple, peeled, cored, and cut into chunks
4 limes, quartered

Cut the pork into 2-inch cubes.

In a 6-quart pot over medium heat, brown the pork in 1 tablespoon oil. Remove from the pan and set aside.

Add the onions and garlic to the pan. Cook for 3 to 4 minutes. Add the stock, coriander, peppers, cornmeal, and pepper flakes. Bring to a boil, cover the pan, reduce the heat, and simmer for 15 minutes. Transfer to a blender or food processor and puree until smooth.

Return the mixture to the pan. Add the pork, cover, and simmer over low heat for 1 hour, or until the pork is very tender.

Cut the chicken into 1-inch pieces. Add to the pan. Simmer for 20 minutes.

Cut the bananas in half lengthwise, then in half crosswise.

In a large nonstick frying pan, heat the remaining 1 tablespoon oil. Add the bananas and cook until lightly browned on each side.

To serve, spoon the meat mixture onto a large platter. Sprinkle with the pumpkin seeds. Surround with the bananas, pineapples, and limes. To eat, squeeze lime juice over the food as you go.

Serves 6

LONDON BROIL
WITH GARLIC MARINADE

◇ *Per serving*

294 calories
6.9 g. fat
(21% of calories)
2.7 g. dietary fiber
70 mg. cholesterol
47 mg. sodium

12 ounces lean top round, ¾ inch thick
⅓ cup red-wine vinegar
3 cloves garlic, minced
3 bay leaves
2 teaspoons olive oil
4 potatoes, steamed or microwaved

*T*rim all visible fat from the meat, then pierce it with a fork in about a dozen places. Place the meat in shallow baking dish or ovenproof casserole.

In a cup, combine the vinegar, garlic, bay leaves, and oil. Pour over the meat, cover, and refrigerate overnight. Discard the bay leaves.

Transfer the meat to a rack and broil about 5 inches from the heat until cooked through, about 5 minutes on each side for medium rare. Serve with the potatoes.

Serves 4

◇

LAMB MEATBALLS
WITH PEAR-TURNIP PUREE

◇ *Per serving*

531 calories
12.5 g. fat
(21% of calories)
6.8 g. dietary fiber
79 mg. cholesterol
201 mg. sodium

1 pound turnips, thinly sliced
2 large pears, chopped
½ cup chopped scallions
1 tablespoon canola oil
¼ cup crumbled blue cheese
1 teaspoon grated nutmeg
1½ pounds extra-lean ground lamb
1 cup wheat germ
1 onion, minced
¼ cup egg substitute
¼ cup minced fresh parsley
2 teaspoons dried thyme
12 ounces thin noodles

Steam the turnips until tender, about 30 minutes. Add the pears and steam 5 minutes more.

In a small pan, sauté the scallions in the oil until tender. Transfer to a blender or food processor. Add the turnips, pears, 2 tablespoons of the cheese, and nutmeg. Process until well blended. Pour into a 2-quart saucepan and keep warm.

In a large bowl, combine the lamb, wheat germ, onions, egg substitute, parsley, thyme, and remaining cheese. Mix well. Shape into small meatballs.

In a large nonstick frying pan over medium heat, sauté the meatballs until cooked through, about 5 to 10 minutes. Blot on paper towels to remove any excess fat.

Cook the noodles in boiling water until tender. Drain.

Serve the meatballs with the puree and noodles.

Serves 6

◇   ◇   ◇

ORCHARD MEAT LOAF

◇ *Per serving*

209 calories
5 g. fat
(22% of calories)
1.7 g. dietary fiber
54 mg. cholesterol
79 mg. sodium

1¼ pounds extra-lean ground beef
1 cup rolled oats
1 large onion, diced
1 cup shredded apples
½ cup minced fresh parsley
¼ cup egg substitute
1½ teaspoons Worcestershire sauce
½ teaspoon dried basil
½ teaspoon dried oregano
¼ teaspoon hot-pepper sauce

In a large bowl, combine the beef, oats, onions, apples, parsley, egg substitute, Worcestershire, basil, oregano, and hot-pepper sauce.

Coat a 9 × 5-inch loaf pan with nonstick spray. Add the meat mixture. Bake at 350°F for 1 hour.

Serves 6

Stuffed Baked Potatoes

◇ *Per serving*

210 calories
2.8 g. fat
(12% of calories)
3.8 g. dietary fiber
32 mg. cholesterol
66 mg. sodium

4 large potatoes
8 ounces extra-lean ground beef
1 onion, minced
1 sweet red pepper, minced

¼ cup minced fresh parsley
1 teaspoon Dijon mustard
¼ teaspoon dried basil

¼ teaspoon dried thyme
⅛ teaspoon red pepper

*B*ake the potatoes at 375°F for 1 hour, or until easily pierced with a fork.

In a large nonstick frying pan over high heat, brown the beef for 5 minutes. Add the onions, peppers, parsley, mustard, basil, thyme, and red pepper. Cook for 3 minutes. Reserve ½ cup.

Cut a thin slice off the top of each potato. With a spoon, scoop out the insides, leaving a ¼-inch-thick shell. Mash the scooped-out potatoes and add to the beef mixture in the pan.

Spoon the mixture into the shells, mounding it. Sprinkle with the reserved mixture. Reheat in the oven for 5 minutes.

Serves 4

Tomatoes Stuffed with Lamb Hash

◇ *Per serving*

199 calories
3.9 g. fat
(18% of calories)
3 g. dietary fiber
39 mg. cholesterol
279 mg. sodium

1½ cups diced cooked lean lamb
1½ cups diced cooked potatoes
¼ cup snipped chives

1 cup nonfat yogurt
¼ cup nonfat mayonnaise
1 tablespoon vinegar

1 teaspoon dillweed
4 extra-large tomatoes
¼ cup chopped fresh parsley

*I*n a large bowl, combine the lamb, potatoes, and chives.

In a small bowl, whisk together the yogurt, mayonnaise, vinegar, and dill. Pour over the lamb and mix well.

Cut off the tops of the tomatoes. Scoop out the pulp, being careful not to pierce the skins. Mince 1 cup of the tomato pulp and add it to the lamb mixture.

Stuff the tomato shells with the hash. Sprinkle with the parsley.

Serves 4

◇ ◇ ◇

MARINADE MAGIC FOR MEAT

Low-fat meats are tougher than marbleized cuts, but they can be tenderized by a good marinade. Marinades also offer added flavor as the meat absorbs the liquids and spices used in the recipe.

Marinades work best on small pieces of meat. For maximum effect, marinate the meat overnight and turn the pieces frequently to expose as much surface as possible to the marinade's flavorful ingredients. After marinating, broil, bake, grill, or stir-fry the meat.

Since most marinades are acid-based, always use a nonreactive container, such as glass, ceramic, or stainless steel. Don't use aluminum or plastic. And remember that although acidic ingredients help protect the food from bacterial growth, refrigerating the meat during marination is the safest course.

Here are some savory citrus marinades suitable for any type of meat. Vary the proportions to suit your own taste.

- Lemon juice and pulp, dried tarragon, and minced shallots
- Lime juice and pulp, nonfat yogurt, and curry powder
- Lemon juice and pulp and cranberry sauce
- Lemon juice and pulp, crushed fennel seeds, and minced garlic
- Orange juice and pulp, low-sodium soy sauce, minced ginger, and sesame oil
- Lime juice and pulp, peanut oil, and hot-pepper sauce
- Lime juice and pulp and minced fresh ginger
- Lemon juice and pulp, tomato puree, dried oregano, and dried basil
- Lime juice and pulp, grated nutmeg, and ground allspice
- Lemon juice and pulp, coarse mustard, and dried sage

Sizzling Fajitas

◇ *Per serving*

282 calories
7.3 g. fat
(23% of calories)
1.6 g. dietary fiber
68 mg. cholesterol
38 mg. sodium

1 pound top round, trimmed of all visible fat
½ cup lime juice
2 tablespoons minced fresh coriander
2 teaspoons olive oil

1 clove garlic, minced
¾ teaspoon ground cumin
¼ teaspoon dried oregano
¼ teaspoon black pepper
1 cup thinly sliced onions

3 chili peppers, cut into thin strips
1 cup diced tomatoes
6 flour tortillas, warmed

Freeze the beef until firm enough to slice easily, about 30 minutes. Cut across the grain and slightly on the bias into ¼-inch slices.

In a large bowl, combine ¼ cup lime juice, coriander, oil, garlic, cumin, oregano, and black pepper. Add the steak. Cover, refrigerate, and allow to marinate 2 hours, stirring occasionally.

Coat a broiler rack with nonstick spray. With tongs, remove the steak from the marinade (reserve the marinade) and arrange in a single layer on the rack. Broil about 5 inches from the heat for 4 minutes. Turn and broil another 4 minutes, or until lightly browned.

In a large nonstick frying pan over medium-high heat, combine the reserved marinade and the onions and chili peppers. Cook for 3 to 4 minutes, or until crisp-tender.

Add the tomatoes and remaining ¼ cup lime juice. Cook, stirring occasionally, for 3 minutes, or until just heated. Add the meat and toss to combine.

Divide the mixture among the tortillas. Roll to enclose the filling.

Serves 6

PEACHES AND PORK

◇ *Per serving*

337 calories
8.5 g. fat
(23% of calories)
3.3 g. dietary fiber
55 mg. cholesterol
114 mg. sodium

12 ounces pork tenderloin, trimmed of all fat
2 teaspoons cornstarch
¼ cup defatted stock
1 tablespoon peeled minced gingerroot

1 egg white, lightly beaten
3 cloves garlic, minced
1 teaspoon low-sodium soy sauce
½ teaspoon Chinese five-spice powder

1 tablespoon canola oil
2 cups julienned peaches
2 tablespoons toasted pine nuts
3 scallions, minced
2 cups hot cooked rice

*F*reeze the pork until firm enough to slice easily, about 30 minutes. Cut against the grain into thin slices. Sprinkle with the cornstarch.

In a large bowl, combine the stock, ginger, egg white, garlic, soy sauce, and five-spice powder. Add the pork, toss to combine, and allow to marinate for 30 minutes.

In a large nonstick frying pan over medium-high heat, heat 2 teaspoons oil for 1 minute. Add the pork and marinade. Stir-fry for 3 minutes, or until cooked through. Remove the pork from the pan.

Add the remaining 1 teaspoon oil to the pan. Add the peaches and stir-fry for about 30 seconds. Add the pine nuts, scallions, and pork. Stir-fry until heated through. Serve with the rice.

Serves 4

Chutneys are flavorful condiments of Indian origin that are a *must* for the health-conscious kitchen. They add needed pizzazz to no-salt, low-fat cookery. And they're especially good with very lean meats that must be braised a long time to be tender. (They're also delicious with plain poached chicken breasts or steamed fish fillets—foods that need a little extra culinary oomph.)

◇ ───────────────────────────

Fresh Pineapple Chutney

1 pineapple, peeled, cored, and diced	1 green chili pepper, seeded and finely chopped
¼ cup minced fresh coriander	2 tablespoons lime juice
¼ cup minced fresh mint	1 tablespoon peeled grated gingerroot

In a large bowl, mix the pineapple, coriander, mint, peppers, lime juice, and ginger. Cover and let stand for 30 minutes.

Makes about 3 cups

◇*Per ¼ cup:* 21 calories, 0.2 g. fat (9% of calories), 0.5 g. dietary fiber, 0 mg. cholesterol, 1 mg. sodium

◇ ───────────────────────────

Peach Chutney

¼ cup honey	1 tablespoon peeled minced gingerroot
¼ cup white-wine vinegar	¼ teaspoon ground cumin
¼ cup minced onions	1 pound peaches
3 tablespoons raisins, chopped	

In a 2-quart saucepan, combine the honey, vinegar, onions, raisins, ginger, and cumin. Simmer for 10 minutes.

Pit and coarsely chop the peaches. Add to the pan and simmer, stirring occasionally, for 30 minutes, or until thick.

Transfer to a medium bowl. Serve warm or cold. Store tightly covered in the refrigerator.

Makes about 2¼ cups

◇*Per ¼ cup: 63 calories, 0.1 g. fat (1% of calories), 1.1 g. dietary fiber, 0 mg. cholesterol, 2 mg. sodium*

◇ ─────────────────────────────

Apple-Tomato Chutney

2 pounds tomatoes, peeled, seeded, and chopped	2 large apples, coarsely chopped
½ cup minced red onions	¼ cup apple-cider vinegar
½ cup chopped celery	4 allspice berries, crushed
1 bay leaf	½ teaspoon ground cinnamon
1 tablespoon apple juice	

In a medium saucepan, combine the tomatoes, onions, celery, bay leaf, and apple juice. Simmer for 5 minutes.

Add the apples, vinegar, allspice, and cinnamon. Partially cover and simmer, stirring frequently, for 40 minutes, or until thick. Discard the bay leaf.

Transfer to a medium bowl. Serve warm or cold. Store tightly covered in the refrigerator.

Makes about 3 cups

◇*Per ¼ cup: 34 calories, 0.4 g. fat (11% of calories), 1.7 g. dietary fiber, 0 mg. cholesterol, 12 mg. sodium*

BARBECUED BEEF SATAY

◇ *Per serving*

380 calories
5.6 g. fat
(13% of calories)
2.3 g. dietary fiber
65 mg. cholesterol
170 mg. sodium

1 pound top round, trimmed of all visible fat
1 large onion, minced
¼ cup defatted stock
¼ cup lemon juice
1 tablespoon peeled grated gingerroot
2 teaspoons low-sodium soy sauce
1 teaspoon caraway seeds
1 teaspoon ground coriander
½ teaspoon turmeric
½ teaspoon ground red pepper
3 cloves garlic, minced
3–4 cups hot cooked rice

Cut the beef into 1-inch cubes. In a large bowl, combine the beef, onions, stock, lemon juice, ginger, soy sauce, caraway, coriander, turmeric, red pepper, and garlic. Cover and allow to marinate for 2 hours.

Thread the meat onto small skewers. Reserve the marinade and transfer to a 1-quart saucepan.

Broil the meat 4 inches from the heat for 6 minutes, turning once and brushing with marinade.

Boil the marinade for 1 minute.

Serve the meat atop the rice. Spoon on the marinade.

Serves 4

Scallops of Veal
with Fennel and Grapes

◇ *Per serving*

424 calories
10.5 g. fat
(22% of calories)
2.7 g. dietary fiber
92 mg. cholesterol
129 mg. sodium

1 pound veal scallops	½ cup defatted chicken stock
1 tablespoon canola oil	1 fennel bulb, halved lengthwise and thinly sliced
1 tablespoon minced fresh parsley	½ cup minced shallots
½ teaspoon dried savory	2 cups small red grapes
½ teaspoon dried rosemary	8 ounces linguine

*P*at the veal dry with paper towels. Place between sheets of waxed paper and flatten with a mallet until about ⅛ inch thick.

In a cup, combine the oil, parsley, savory, and rosemary. Brush over the veal. cover with plastic and refrigerate for 3 to 4 hours.

Coat a large nonstick frying pan with nonstick spray. Over medium-high heat, sauté the veal in batches for 2 minutes per side, or until slightly browned. Remove to a serving dish and keep warm.

In the same pan, combine the stock, fennel, and shallots. Cook over medium-high heat until the stock is reduced by half and the fennel is tender, about 10 minutes. Add the grapes and heat for 30 seconds. Add the veal; keep warm.

Cook the linguine in boiling water until tender. Drain. Serve with the veal.

Serves 4

MICRO METHOD: Moist Meats

When time's at a premium, remember that you can cook most meats in the microwave. Here's how to get the best results.

- Remember that because microwaving is a moist medium, meats don't stick as they might in a frying pan. Therefore you don't need added fat to prevent sticking.
- Ground meat (choose lean ground top round) cooks wonderfully in the microwave. Although it will not brown, it will render a lot of fat—more fat than broiling, charbroiling, roasting, convection heating, or frying will release. Pour off the fat before adding the meat to a casserole or other dish.
- Lean, thin strips of meat cook more quickly and evenly than thick chunks. For best results, slice the meat against its grain.
- If you're cooking meat without a sauce, don't cover it. That way you won't steam the meat and toughen the protein.
- Microwave pork to an internal temperature of 170° F. Check it with a meat thermometer when you remove the meat from the oven.
- When converting a conventional recipe that calls for a good deal of liquid or a long baking time, reduce the liquid by one-third. Liquid doesn't evaporate during microwaving the way it does on the stove or in the oven. Check the dish as it cooks and add more liquid if necessary to achieve the desired consistency. But be aware that dry foods, such as uncooked rice or pasta, will absorb moisture as they cook; so don't reduce the liquid in the recipes.
- Because microwaving can intensify the flavors of certain seasonings, cut back on herbs and spices before cooking. Taste the dish after microwaving and season it then.
- If you're increasing or decreasing a casserole recipe, try to choose a baking dish that will maintain the ingredients at the same depth as they were in the original recipe. In other words, if you're halving a recipe, choose a proportionately smaller dish. But make sure it's deep enough to prevent boil-overs.

lean meats

Mexican Picadillo

◇ *Per serving*

258 calories
5.4 g. fat
(19% of calories)
3.7 g. dietary fiber
65 mg. cholesterol
78 mg. sodium

1½ pounds extra-lean ground beef
2 onions, minced
1 green pepper, minced
3 cloves garlic, minced
1 cup tomato sauce
2 apples, finely chopped
⅓ cup raisins
2 teaspoons dried oregano
2 teaspoons ground cumin
1 head romaine lettuce
1 lime, cut into wedges

*I*n a large nonstick frying pan over medium heat, brown the beef, breaking it up with a wooden spoon. As soon as the meat begins to lose its pink color, add the onions, peppers, and garlic. Cook, stirring often, until beef has browned and the onions are translucent. Drain any accumulated fat.

Add the tomato sauce, apples, raisins, oregano, and cumin. Cover and simmer for 30 minutes.

Transfer to a large platter. Surround with romaine leaves.

To eat, spoon some meat onto a lettuce leaf, squeeze on some lime juice, then roll up the leaf like a tortilla.

Serves 6

PEAR AND PORK STIR-FRY

◇ *Per serving*

177 calories
4.8 g. fat
(24% of calories)
2.7 g. dietary fiber
56 mg. cholesterol
156 mg. sodium

12 ounces pork tenderloin, trimmed of all visible fat

2 tablespoons defatted chicken stock

2 teaspoons low-sodium soy sauce

1 teaspoon vinegar

1 teaspoon cornstarch

⅛ teaspoon ground cinnamon

2 teaspoons canola oil

2 scallions, shredded

2 tablespoons peeled minced gingerroot

1 clove garlic, minced

2 large pears, sliced ¼ inch thick

1 cup shredded spinach

*F*reeze the pork until firm enough to slice easily, about 30 minutes. Slice across the grain into thin slices. Cut into 1-inch by 2-inch pieces.

In a large bowl, combine the stock, soy sauce, vinegar, cornstarch, and cinnamon. Add the pork and toss gently. Cover and let stand 20 minutes.

In a large nonstick frying pan over medium-high heat, heat the oil for 2 minutes. Add the scallions, ginger, and garlic. Stir-fry for 10 seconds, or until the scallions are translucent.

Add the pork and marinade. Stir-fry until the pork begins to brown, 2 to 3 minutes.

Add the pears and stir-fry 1 minute. Add the spinach. Cook until the spinach begins to wilt, about 1 minute.

Serves 4

Fruited Lamb Curry

½ cup raisins
½ cup hot water
4 potatoes, cubed
2 tablespoons canola oil
1 large onion, chopped
2 tart apples, diced

1 banana, diced
2 cloves garlic, minced
1 tablespoon curry powder
6 ounces tomato paste

1 cup defatted chicken stock
1 bay leaf
12 ounces lamb loin, trimmed of all visible fat

*I*n a cup, soak the raisins in the water for 15 to 30 minutes, until plump.

Steam the potatoes until just tender.

In a 3-quart saucepan over medium heat, heat 1 tablespoon oil. Add the onions. Sauté until transparent, about 5 minutes.

Add the apples, bananas, garlic, and curry powder. Cook, stirring often, until the apple is soft, about 3 minutes. Transfer to a blender or food processor. Add the tomato paste and stock. Blend well.

Return the mixture to the saucepan. Add the potatoes, bay leaf, and raisins (including the soaking water).

Simmer over low heat, stirring, for 10 minutes.

Cut the lamb into ½-inch cubes.

In a large nonstick frying pan over high heat, heat the remaining 1 tablespoon oil. Add the lamb and brown it quickly over high heat until cooked through. Add the lamb to the sauce. Discard the bay leaf.

Serves 4

CHAPTER TWELVE ◇

Vegetable Side Dishes

*F*rom asparagus to zucchini, vegetables add a hefty dose of low-fat flavor to any meal. And while family members may square off over their favorites, all are bound to find something they like.

You might say green and orange are the official colors of the vegetable class. Dark green and orange vegetables such as kale, Swiss chard, carrots, and sweet potatoes get their vibrant hues from carotenoids, plant forms of cancer-fighting vitamin A. These foods add eye appeal as well as delicious flavor to everyday meals.

All the recipes in this chapter aim to help you see your old favorite vegetables in a new light. Instead of serving plain peas or carrots, for example, try Sesame Snow Peas or Carrot Fritters. Instead of buttered green beans, serve Chinese Beans with Sesame Seeds. And as a change of pace from eggplant parmesan, help yourself to Hunan Eggplant, yet another Oriental dream.

Cruciferous vegetables such as brussels sprouts really shine when dressed up in mushroom glaze. And Marinated Cauliflower is a new way to savor another cancer-fighting crucifer. What about those root vegetables—such as parsnips, rutabagas, and turnips—that you may have passed by until now? We've got tantalizing recipes for them, too, such as Far Eastern Rutabagas, Creamed Turnips, and Carrots and Parsnips.

So bring on the vegetables, and don't be surprised if people who used to turn up their noses at vegetables start asking for seconds!

CARROT FRITTERS

◇ *Per serving*

57 calories
1.3 g. fat
(21% of calories)
2 g. dietary fiber
0 mg. cholesterol
67 mg. sodium

¼ cup egg
  substitute
1 tablespoon flour
2 cups shredded
  carrots
2 scallions,
  minced

2 tablespoons
  minced
  parsley
½ teaspoon
  dried tarragon

2 egg whites
1 teaspoon
  olive oil

*I*n a large bowl, combine the egg substitute and flour. Stir in the carrots, scallions, parsley, and tarragon.

In a separate bowl, whip the egg whites with clean beaters until stiff. Fold into the carrot mixture.

Heat the oil on a nonstick griddle. Drop ¼-cup mounds of batter onto the hot griddle. Flatten a bit with the back of a spatula. Fry on both sides until golden brown.

Serves 4

◇   ◇   ◇

CARROTS AND PARSNIPS

◇ *Per serving*

159 calories
0.7 g. fat
(4% of calories)
8.6 g. dietary fiber
0 mg. cholesterol
51 mg. sodium

1 pound carrots,
  chopped
1 pound
  parsnips,
  chopped

1 ripe pear,
  chopped
2 tablespoons
  minced fresh
  chervil or
  parsley

*I*n a 3-quart saucepan, steam the carrots and parsnips until tender, about 10 minutes. Reserve the steaming liquid.

Transfer the carrots and parsnips to a food processor. Add the pears. Puree until smooth, adding just enough cooking liquid to facilitate blending.

Reheat gently before serving. Stir in the chervil or parsley.

Serves 8

Garden-Puff Potatoes

◇ *Per serving*

148 calories
0.6 g. fat
(4% of calories)
5.2 g. dietary fiber
1 mg. cholesterol
53 mg. sodium

4 large baking
  potatoes
1½ cups bite-size
  broccoli
  florets
½ cup diced
  green
  peppers

¼ cup diced
  onions
1 cup shredded
  carrots
⅓ cup
  buttermilk

2 teaspoons
  dillweed
1 tablespoon
  snipped
  chives

Bake the potatoes at 375°F for 1 hour, or until easily pierced with a fork.

Steam the broccoli for 3 minutes. Add the peppers and onions. Steam for 2 minutes.

Cut a thin slice off the top of each potato. Scoop out the pulp, leaving a ¼-inch shell. Reserve the shells and transfer the pulp to a blender.

Add the carrots, buttermilk, and dill. Whip on high speed for 5 minutes, or until light and fluffy. Add more buttermilk, if needed.

Transfer to a medium bowl. Fold in the steamed vegetables.

Spoon the potato mixture into the reserved shells. Broil about 4 inches from the heat for 5 minutes, or until lightly browned. Sprinkle with the chives.

Serves 4

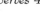

Far Eastern Rutabagas

◇ *Per serving*

109 calories
2.7 g. fat
(23% of calories)
10.5 g. dietary fiber

2 pounds
  rutabagas
1 tablespoon
  low-sodium
  soy sauce
1½ teaspoons
  canola oil

½ teaspoon
  sesame oil
2 cloves garlic,
  minced
¼ teaspoon red
  pepper

¼ cup thinly
  sliced
  scallions

0 mg. cholesterol
196 mg. sodium

*P*eel the rutabagas and cut into ½-inch chunks. Place in a 3-quart saucepan, cover with cold water, and cook over medium heat until tender, about 20 to 25 minutes. Drain. Return to the pan and stir over medium heat until all the excess moisture evaporates, about 2 minutes.

In a large frying pan, combine the soy sauce, canola oil, sesame oil, garlic, and pepper. Heat for 4 minutes. Add the rutabagas and toss to combine. Heat for 2 minutes. Sprinkle with the scallions.

Serves 4

GREEN BEANS AND PEPPERS

◇ *Per serving*

142 calories
4 g. fat
(25% of calories)
5 g. dietary fiber
0 mg. cholesterol
61 mg. sodium

12 ounces small red potatoes	⅓ cup tarragon vinegar	½ teaspoon dried marjoram
8 ounces green beans	1 tablespoon olive oil	¼ teaspoon black pepper
2 sweet red peppers	1 teaspoon Dijon mustard	¼ teaspoon Worcestershire sauce
8 cooked artichoke hearts, halved	1 clove garlic, minced	

*S*team the potatoes until tender, about 15 minutes. Cool to warm and slice thinly. Place in a large bowl.

Blanch the beans in boiling water for 5 minutes. Drain and add to the bowl.

Broil the peppers until charred on all sides. Let cool slightly, then peel, seed, and dice. Add to the bowl.

Add the artichokes and toss to combine.

In a small bowl, whisk together the vinegar, oil, mustard, garlic, marjoram, black pepper, and Worcestershire.

Pour over the vegetables and toss to combine.

Serves 4

FRESH TALK ABOUT VEGETABLES

Safeguard the nutrients in your produce by choosing and storing your selections properly.

Vegetable	Look for	Storage
Asparagus	Firm, smooth, round spears; closed, compact tips; rich green color	Wrap stems in moist toweling; refrigerate in plastic bags; will keep 2–3 days
Broccoli	Small, closed buds with no trace of yellow; moderate size; firm yet tender stems and branches	Refrigerate in plastic bags; will keep 3–5 days
Corn	Moist, green husks; bright, plump kernels	Refrigerate in husks; will keep 1–2 days
Eggplant	Firm, heavy body; small blossom-end scar; rich purple color; shiny, tight, smooth skin	Store in cool place or in refrigerator; put in plastic bag to retain moisture; will keep 2–4 days
Lima beans	Well-filled, clean, shiny green pods	Refrigerate in shells; will keep 2–5 days
Peas	Crisp, bright green pods filled but not bulging with peas	Refrigerate uncovered in pods; will keep 2–4 days
Snap beans	Crisp, long, slender pods; seeds less than half grown; good color	Refrigerate in plastic bags; will keep 2–5 days
Snow or sugar snap peas	Crisp, slender, bright green pods with immature peas	Refrigerate in plastic bags; will keep 1–2 days
Summer squash	Firm, glossy, tender skin; fairly heavy for size; slender	Refrigerate in plastic bags; will keep 3–5 days
Tomatoes	Firm, plump bodies with uniform color; small blossom-end scar	Ripen and store at room temperature; will keep at least 1 week

CHRISTMAS CABBAGE

2 pounds cabbage, chopped into ½-inch pieces
1 tart apple, cubed
1 pear, cubed
1 large onion, diced
1 navel orange, sectioned and chopped
¼ cup defatted stock
1 tablespoon
1½ teaspoons peeled minced gingerroot
1 tablespoon red-wine vinegar
1 tablespoon all-fruit marmalade

*I*n a 4-quart pot, combine the cabbage, apples, pears, onions, oranges, stock, honey, and ginger. Cover and simmer, stirring occasionally, for 30 minutes. Add the vinegar and marmalade. Cook for 5 minutes.

Serves 6

◇   ◇   ◇

FRENCH-STYLE CHARD

4 cups coarsely shredded Swiss chard
2 cloves garlic, minced
¼ cup defatted chicken stock
2 tablespoons grated Sapsago or Parmesan cheese

*I*n a large nonstick frying pan, sauté the chard and garlic in the stock until wilted, about 5 minutes. Sprinkle with the cheese.

Serves 4

SWEET-CORN FRITTERS

1 cup nonfat yogurt
½ cup applesauce
1 cup corn
½ cup egg substitute
¼ cup skim milk

⅓ cup unbleached flour
½ teaspoon baking powder
2 tablespoons snipped chives

¼ teaspoon dried oregano
1 tablespoon canola oil

*L*ine a strainer with cheesecloth or a coffee filter. Place over a bowl. Spoon in the yogurt and allow to drain for 30 minutes.

Transfer to a small bowl. Whisk in the applesauce. Set aside.

In a food processor, chop the corn with on/off turns until crushed but not pureed. Transfer to a medium bowl. Stir in the egg substitute and milk.

Add the flour, baking powder, chives, and oregano. If the batter is too thick, stir in additional milk.

Heat a large nonstick frying pan over medium heat. Brush lightly with oil. Drop batter by heaping teaspoonfuls into the pan. Cook the fritters until golden brown on both sides, about 4 minutes. Repeat, brushing the pan with additional oil, until all the batter is used.

Serve the fritters with the applesauce mixture.

Serves 4

◇ ◇ ◇

GREENS WITH GARLIC

⅓ cup defatted chicken stock
8 cloves unpeeled garlic
1 pound kale, shredded

2 tablespoons lemon juice
2 tablespoons tomato juice
1 teaspoon olive oil

½ teaspoon red-pepper flakes
8 slices French bread

vegetable side dishes

0 mg. cholesterol
469 mg. sodium

*I*n an ovenproof custard cup, combine the stock and garlic. Bake at 350°F, stirring occasionally, until the garlic is soft, about 30 minutes.

Steam the kale until just tender, about 4 minutes.

In a large bowl whisk together the lemon juice, tomato juice, oil, and pepper flakes. Add the kale and toss to coat.

To serve, peel each clove of garlic and spread on a slice of bread. Mound the greens on the bread.

Serves 4

CREAMED TURNIPS

◇ *Per serving*

89 calories
0.8 g. fat
(8% of calories)
4.3 g. dietary fiber
2 mg. cholesterol
130 mg. sodium

2 pounds small turnips
1 cup thinly sliced onions
1½ tablespoons unbleached flour
1 cup skim milk

¼ teaspoon dried thyme
¼ teaspoon grated nutmeg
⅛ teaspoon black pepper

2 tablespoons shredded low-fat Swiss cheese

*P*eel and quarter the turnips. Steam the turnips and onions until the turnips are tender, about 10 minutes. Transfer to a large bowl.

In a 1-quart saucepan, whisk the flour with about 2 tablespoons of milk until smooth. Whisk in the remaining milk. Cook over medium heat, whisking constantly, until thickened. Add the thyme, nutmeg, and pepper.

Pour the sauce over the turnips and mix well.

Coat a 1½-quart casserole with nonstick spray. Add the turnip mixture. Sprinkle with the cheese.

Bake at 350°F for 15 minutes.

Serves 4

Oriental Gingered Vegetables

◇ *Per serving*

60 calories
1.6 g. fat
(24% of calories)
3.3 g. dietary fiber
0 mg. cholesterol
173 mg. sodium

1 cup sliced green beans
1 cup broccoli florets
1 cup thinly sliced carrots
1 cup sliced asparagus
1 cup thinly sliced mushrooms
½ cup julienned sweet red peppers
1 tablespoon peeled minced gingerroot
1 clove garlic, minced
1 teaspoon canola oil
1 tablespoon low-sodium soy sauce

Steam the beans, broccoli, carrots, and asparagus until crisp-tender, about 5 minutes.

In a large nonstick frying pan over medium-high heat, sauté the mushrooms, peppers, ginger, and garlic in the oil until light brown, about 3 minutes.

Add the steamed vegetables and soy sauce. Stir-fry for 1 to 2 minutes.

Serves 4

Tomato and Zucchini Gratin

◇ *Per serving*

295 calories
6 g. fat
(18% of calories)
4.3 g. dietary fiber

1 large onion, thinly sliced
1 tablespoon olive oil
1 pound zucchini, thinly sliced
¼ teaspoon dried thyme
¼ teaspoon dried basil
3 cups cooked rice
1 large tomato, thinly sliced
¼ cup grated Parmesan cheese

5 mg. cholesterol
126 mg. sodium

In a large frying pan over medium heat, sauté the onions in the oil for 2 minutes. Add the zucchini and sauté until tender, about 4 minutes. Stir in the thyme and basil. Remove from the heat.

Coat a 1½-quart casserole with nonstick spray. Layer half of the rice in the dish. Top with half of the zucchini and half of the tomatoes. Sprinkle with half of the cheese. Repeat.

Bake at 375°F for 15 minutes, or until heated through and lightly browned.

Serves 4

◇   ◇   ◇

Savoy Puree in Potato Shells

◇ *Per serving*

187 calories
5.2 g. fat
(25% of calories)
5.6 g. dietary fiber
0 mg. cholesterol
45 mg. sodium

4 large baking potatoes	1½ tablespoons olive oil	½ teaspoon dried chervil
1 pound savoy cabbage, shredded	¼ cup minced fresh parsley	¼ teaspoon ground black pepper

Bake the potatoes at 375°F for 1 hour, or until easily pierced with a fork.

In a large frying pan, combine the cabbage and oil. Cover and cook over low heat, stirring frequently, until caramelized and very tender, about 40 minutes.

Cut a thin slice off the top of each potato. Scoop out the pulp, leaving a ¼-inch shell. Reserve the shells and transfer the pulp to a large bowl. Mash well. Add the cabbage, parsley, chervil, and pepper.

Spoon into the potato shells.

Serves 4

Moroccan Carrot Salad

◇ *Per serving*

72 calories
2 g. fat
(25% of calories)
3.8 g. dietary fiber
0 mg. cholesterol
42 mg. sodium

1 pound carrots, julienned
2 cloves garlic, minced
1 scallion, minced
2 tablespoons minced fresh parsley
2 teaspoons dillweed
2 tablespoons lemon juice
1½ teaspoons olive oil
½ teaspoon ground cumin
¼ teaspoon paprika
⅛ teaspoon ground cinnamon
⅛ teaspoon red pepper

Steam the carrots and garlic for 5 minutes, until crisp-tender. Transfer to a large bowl. Add the scallions, parsley, and dill.

In a small bowl, whisk together the lemon juice, oil, cumin, paprika, cinnamon, and red pepper. Pour over the carrots and mix well. Refrigerate until cold.

Serves 4

◇   ◇   ◇

Chinese Beans with Sesame Seeds

◇ *Per serving*

136 calories
3.7 g. fat
(24% of calories)
3.4 g. dietary fiber
0 mg. cholesterol
111 mg. sodium

12 ounces green beans
3 tablespoons rice-wine vinegar
1 teaspoon canola oil
2 teaspoons low-sodium soy sauce
1 teaspoon honey
1 tablespoon peeled minced gingerroot
1 tablespoon snipped chives
1 clove garlic, minced
⅛ teaspoon red pepper
4 scallions, sliced diagonally
1 sweet red or yellow pepper, cut into strips
3 tablespoons toasted sesame seeds
2 cups steamed cubed potatoes

*I*f the beans are young and small, leave them whole. Otherwise, snap in half or slice lengthwise. Blanch in boiling water for 2 to 3 minutes. Drain and rinse under cold water.

In a small bowl, whisk together the vinegar, oil, soy sauce, and honey. Stir in the ginger, chives, garlic, and red pepper.

In a large nonstick frying pan over medium-high heat, heat 1 tablespoon of the dressing. Add the beans and toss to coat. Cover and cook for 3 to 4 minutes, or until crisp-tender.

Transfer to a serving platter. Top with the scallions and sliced peppers. Lightly drizzle with the dressing and sprinkle with the sesame seeds. Serve with the potatoes.

Serves 4

◇   ◇   ◇

STIR-FRY WITH SNOW PEAS, CELERY, AND PISTACHIOS

◇ *Per serving*

34 calories
0.9 g. fat
(24% of calories)
1.9 g. dietary fiber
0 mg. cholesterol
35 mg. sodium

1 cup sliced celery
¼ cup minced scallions
¼ cup defatted chicken stock

1 cup snow peas
1 teaspoon dried thyme
¼ teaspoon black pepper

2 teaspoons chopped pistachios
¼ cup minced fresh parsley

*I*n a 1-quart saucepan, cook the celery in water to cover until crisp-tender, about 3 to 5 minutes. Drain.

In a large nonstick frying pan over medium heat, cook the scallions in the stock until light brown, about 5 minutes. Add the celery, snow peas, thyme, and pepper. Cook for several minutes. Remove from the heat and add the pistachios and parsley.

Serves 4

Brussels Sprouts
with Mushroom Glaze

◇ *Per serving*

67 calories
1.1 g. fat
(15% of calories)
5.1 g. dietary fiber
<1 mg. cholesterol
74 mg. sodium

| 1 pound brussels sprouts | 2 teaspoons lemon juice | 1 teaspoon dried thyme |
| 1 cup defatted beef stock | 2 teaspoons Dijon mustard | 1 cup thinly sliced mushrooms |

*T*rim the brussels sprouts and halve lengthwise. Steam until tender, about 10 minutes. Set aside.

In a large nonstick frying pan over medium-high heat, bring the stock to a boil. Whisk in the lemon juice, mustard, and thyme. Add the mushrooms. Boil until the stock is reduced by half, about 5 minutes. Add the brussels sprouts. Toss well to coat with the glaze.

Serves 4

HOT-TOPPED POTATOES

Spuds are a health watcher's dream: high in nutrients and low in fat. Just don't cancel out their healthy qualities with a blanket of butter, sour cream, or bacon bits. Instead try these tasty low-fat toppings.

■ Chopped tomatoes, mashed pinto beans, minced jalapeño peppers, and melted low-fat Monterey Jack cheese

■ Stir-fried sweet red peppers, sliced mushrooms, and snow peas flavored with minced ginger and garlic

■ Chopped steamed asparagus, toasted pine nuts, and blenderized low-fat cottage cheese

■ Sliced wild mushrooms, shredded spinach, and minced garlic sautéed in olive oil and sprinkled with grated Sapsago or Parmesan cheese

■ Toasted walnuts, chopped red onion, chopped black olives, and a sprinkling of crumbled feta cheese

Maple Sweet Potatoes

4 large sweet
  potatoes
¼ cup nonfat
  yogurt

3 tablespoons
  maple syrup
3 tablespoons
  orange juice

*B*ake the potatoes at 375°F for 1¼ hours, or until easily pierced with a fork. Slice in half lengthwise. Scoop out the pulp, leaving a ¼-inch shell. Reserve the shells and transfer the pulp to a large bowl.

Mash the pulp and stir in the yogurt, maple syrup, and orange juice. Spoon the filling into the reserved shells.

Return to the oven and bake for 5 minutes to heat through.

Serves 4

◇　　　　　　　　◇　　　　　　　　◇

Spicy Roasted Potatoes

1 tablespoon
  coarse mustard
1 tablespoon
  olive oil
1 clove garlic,
  minced

1 teaspoon
  dried tarragon
¼ teaspoon
  paprika

⅛ teaspoon red
  pepper
2 large baking
  potatoes

*I*n a medium bowl, mix the mustard, oil, garlic, tarragon, paprika, and red pepper into a smooth paste.

Cut the potatoes into 1-inch pieces. Pat dry with paper towels. Add to the bowl and toss to coat.

Coat a baking sheet with nonstick spray. Add the potatoes in a single layer. Bake at 425°F for 30 to 35 minutes, or until tender.

Serves 4

Rosemary Asparagus

◇ *Per serving*

44 calories
0.7 g. fat
(14% of calories)
2.6 g. dietary fiber
0 mg. cholesterol
23 mg. sodium

1 cup defatted chicken stock
1 clove garlic, halved
1 teaspoon dried rosemary

1 bay leaf
1 pound thin asparagus spears
½ cup chopped onions

1 tablespoon minced fresh parsley

*P*our the stock into a large frying pan. Add the garlic, rosemary, and bay leaf. Bring to a simmer.

Prepare the asparagus by holding each spear at its ends and bending until it snaps. Discard the tough bottom part. Set the spears in the frying pan and cover with the onions. Partially cover the pan. Simmer for 4 minutes.

Remove the spears from the stock and place on a serving platter. Discard the bay leaf. Strain the stock into a small bowl, reserving the onions and garlic.

Place the onions, garlic, and parsley in a blender or food processor. Add ⅓ cup of the reserved stock. Process until smooth. Drizzle the sauce over the warm asparagus.

Serves 4

◇   ◇   ◇

Beets with Pecans and Dill

◇ *Per serving*

163 calories
4.4 g. fat
(24% of calories)
6.6 g. dietary fiber

2 pounds beets
1 pound onions, thinly sliced
⅓ cup defatted chicken stock
½ cup minced shallots

¼ cup minced fresh parsley
2 tablespoons chopped pecans
1½ teaspoons olive oil

½ teaspoon black pepper
¼ teaspoon dillweed

0 mg. cholesterol
114 mg. sodium

In a 3-quart saucepan, cook the beets in water to cover until easily pierced with a skewer, about 50 minutes. Drain and plunge into cold water. Trim off the tops and slip off the skins. Thinly slice the beets crosswise.

In a large frying pan, combine the onions and stock. Cover and cook over medium heat until very soft, about 20 minutes. Add the shallots and cook for 5 minutes.

In a cup, combine the parsley, pecans, oil, pepper, and dill.

Coat a 9 × 9-inch baking dish with nonstick spray. Add one-fourth of the beets in a single layer. Top with one-third of the onions. Sprinkle with one-third of the parsley mixture.

Repeat two times. End with a layer of beets.

Cover the dish with foil. Bake at 325°F for 35 to 45 minutes.

Serves 4

◇

HUNAN EGGPLANT

◇ *Per serving*

86 calories
2.4 g. fat
(25% of calories)
2.6 g. dietary fiber
0 mg. cholesterol
55 mg. sodium

1½ pounds eggplant	2 cloves garlic, minced	1 teaspoon honey
1 teaspoon canola oil	1 tablespoon lemon juice	1 teapoon sesame oil
1 teaspoon peeled minced gingerroot	1 teaspoon low-sodium soy sauce	

Slice the eggplant into 1-inch chunks. Steam until tender, about 12 minutes.

In a large nonstick frying pan over medium heat, heat the canola oil. Add the ginger and garlic. Sauté until fragrant, about 3 minutes. Stir in the lemon juice, soy sauce, honey, and sesame oil.

Add the eggplant and toss to coat.

Serves 4

Sesame Snow Peas

◇ *Per serving*

58 calories
1.6 g. fat
(25% of calories)
3.1 g. dietary fiber
0 mg. cholesterol
10 mg. sodium

12	ounces snow peas	½	teaspoon sesame oil
1	carrot, julienned	½	teaspoon grated orange rind
1	tablespoon toasted sesame seeds		

Steam the snow peas and carrots until tender, about 4 minutes.

Transfer to a medium bowl. Add the sesame seeds, oil, and orange rind. Toss to combine.

Serves 4

◇ ◇ ◇

Vegetable Egg Roll-Ups

◇ *Per serving*

77 calories
2 g. fat
(23% of calories)
2.5 g. dietary fiber
0 mg. cholesterol
70 mg. sodium

1½	teaspoons olive oil	1	cup mung bean sprouts	4	egg whites
1	cup shredded carrots	1	cup sliced mushrooms	1	small head Boston lettuce
1	cup thinly sliced onions				

In a large nonstick frying pan over medium-high heat, heat the oil. Add the carrots and onions. Stir-fry for 3 minutes.

Add the sprouts and mushrooms. Stir-fry for 3 minutes.

In a cup, whisk the egg whites with a fork until frothy. Add to the vegetables. Stir slowly with a fork until the whites are cooked, about 1 minute.

Separate the lettuce into individual leaves. Divide the vegetable mixture evenly among the lettuce. Loosely roll up the leaves and eat with your hands.

Serves 4

vegetable side dishes

MARINATED CAULIFLOWER

◇ *Per serving*

110 calories
2.8 g. fat
(23% of calories)
6.9 g. dietary fiber
0 mg. cholesterol
38 mg. sodium

1 head cauliflower
2 red onions, thinly sliced
2 teaspoons olive oil
1 tablespoon white-wine vinegar

1 tablespoon lemon juice
3 tablespoons minced fresh parsley
2 cloves garlic, minced

½ teaspoon dillweed
¼ teaspoon dried thyme

*B*reak the cauliflower into florets. Steam the cauliflower and onions until tender, about 5 minutes.

In a large bowl, whisk together the oil, vinegar, and lemon juice. Stir in the parsley, garlic, dill, and thyme.

Refrigerate for several hours, turning the vegetables in the marinade occasionally.

Serves 4

CHAPTER THIRTEEN ◇

Grand Finales

The perfect "grand finale" finishes off a healthy meal with its own positive contributions. It never sabotages a good diet with an overload of sugar, fat, or calories. That's why the accent is on sweet, succulent fruits and other healthy ingredients in this dessert chapter.

The very best desserts, of course, are juicy, vine-ripened fruits savored all by themselves. And we encourage you to choose these healthy sweets for everyday enjoyment. But when you hanker for a special indulgence, appease your sweet tooth the *right* way—with nutrient-dense desserts. Reach for a fruit-based sweet, such as Spiced Apples or Peach Soufflé. They're easy as pie and delightfully lean.

Speaking of pie, choosing a single-crust tart cuts fat and calories. For extra measure, replace the saturated butter, lard, or hydrogenated shortening in standard recipes with healthy canola oil. Then pile the shell high with pectin-rich fruit, as in Apple Tart or Pear-Cheese Pie. Or have your pie without a crust as in Lemon Pumpkin Pie. For variety, make a Berry Custard that tastes rich and creamy but is very low in fat and cholesterol.

For warm-weather enjoyment, choose summer-ripe fruits for easy desserts such as Strawberries with Two Melons or Nectarines with Sauce Cardinale. In winter, take advantage of dried or tropical fruit and whip up Marinated Figs and Apricots or a wonderful Tropical Compote.

With desserts like the ones in this chapter, you can eat up and safeguard your health. Enjoy!

PEAR-CHEESE PIE

◇ *Per serving*

299 calories
6.5 g. fat
(20% of calories)
5.6 g. dietary fiber
3 mg. cholesterol
279 mg. sodium

2 cups whole wheat flour
3 tablespoons oil
⅓ cup ice water
3 cups thinly sliced pears
2 cups low-fat cottage cheese
1 cup egg substitute
¼ cup honey
1 tablespoon orange juice
2 teaspoons unbleached flour
¼ teaspoon ground cinnamon
1 teaspoon vanilla extract
¼ teaspoon almond extract
1 tablespoon lemon juice
2 cups apple juice
3 tablespoons orange marmalade

*P*lace the flour in a medium bowl. Drizzle with the oil and mix well. Sprinkle on the water and mix until you can form the dough into a ball. Roll into an 11-inch circle. Fit into a 9-inch pie plate. Crimp the edges.

Arrange 1 cup of the pears in the pie shell.

In a food processor, puree the cottage cheese until smooth. Add the egg substitute, honey, orange juice, flour, cinnamon, vanilla, and almond extract. Mix well. Pour into the pie shell.

Bake at 350°F for 15 minutes. Reduce the temperature to 325°F and bake another 45 minutes, or until the filling is set.

In a large bowl, combine the remaining pears and the lemon juice. In a large frying pan, bring the apple juice to a boil. Add the pears and cook for 1 minute, stirring constantly. Remove with a slotted spoon and drain well on paper towels.

Arrange the pears in a circle around the edge of the crust, overlapping the slices slightly.

In a 1-quart saucepan, melt the marmalade over low heat. Brush the pears with the marmalade. Chill the pie at least 4 hours.

Serves 8

LEMON PUMPKIN PIE

◇ *Per serving*

95 calories
0.1 g. fat
(<1% of calories)
0.6 g. dietary fiber
2 mg. cholesterol
78 mg. sodium

1½ cups pumpkin puree
¾ cup egg substitute
¾ cup evaporated skim milk
⅓ cup maple syrup

½ teaspoon ground cinnamon
½ teaspoon ground ginger
¼ teaspoon grated nutmeg

1 cup nonfat vanilla yogurt
1 tablespoon lemon juice
2 teaspoons grated lemon rind

Coat a 9-inch plate with nonstick spray.

In a large bowl, beat together the pumpkin, egg substitute, milk, maple syrup, cinnamon, ginger, and nutmeg.

Pour into the pie plate and bake at 350°F for 55 minutes, or until a knife inserted near the center comes out clean. Cool on a wire rack.

In a small bowl, whisk together the yogurt, lemon juice, and lemon rind. Spread on top of the pie. Chill.

Serves 8

◇   ◇   ◇

CHEESECAKE TART

◇ *Per serving*

173 calories
4.5 g. fat
(23% of calories)
2.5 g. dietary fiber
3 mg. cholesterol
267 mg. sodium

CRUST
1 cup crushed nonfat granola
2 tablespoons canola oil
2 tablespoons maple syrup
CHEESECAKE
2 cups low-fat cottage cheese

½ cup egg substitute
¼ cup maple syrup
1 teaspoon vanilla extract
¼ teaspoon almond extract

2 tangerines, sectioned
2 kiwifruit, sliced

To make the crust: Lightly oil a 9-inch tart pan with removable bottom.

In a small bowl, combine the granola, oil, and maple syrup. Press the mixture in the bottom and up the sides of the tart pan.

To make the cheesecake: In a food processor, combine the cottage cheese, egg substitute, maple syrup, vanilla, and almond extract until smooth.

Spoon the filling into the pan. Bake at 325°F for 30 minutes, or until firm.

Let cool on a wire rack. Then chill for at least 3 hours. Top with the tangerines and kiwis before serving.

Serves 8

◇   ◇   ◇

STRAWBERRIES WITH TWO MELONS

◇ *Per serving*

117 calories
0.6 g. fat
(5% of calories)
3.1 g. dietary fiber
1 mg. cholesterol
48 mg. sodium

1½ cups cantaloupe chunks
1½ cups honeydew chunks
2 cups halved strawberries
1 lime, thinly sliced
1 cup nonfat vanilla yogurt
1 tablespoon lime juice
¼ teaspoon ground cardamom

*I*n a large bowl, combine the cantaloupe, honeydew, strawberries, and lime.

In a small bowl, combine the yogurt, lime juice, and cardamom. Pour over the fruit and toss to combine.

Serves 4

MICRO METHOD: Bring Out the Best

Recapture the just-picked sweetness of sun-ripened fruit by microwaving it briefly. Some suggestions:
- Accentuate the flavor of strawberries, raspberries, pineapple, apricots, figs, peaches, nectarines, and other summer fruit by microwaving until just barely warm. Exact time will depend on the quantity, size, and temperature of the fruit. For instance, 10 large room-temperature strawberries (arrange in a circle with tips pointing in) will take about 10 to 20 seconds.
- Get more juice from citrus fruit. Before cutting and squeezing (or eating out of hand), microwave a whole lemon, lime, orange, or tangerine on full power for 15 to 35 seconds, until just slightly warm to the touch. If using the fruit for juice, roll it on the kitchen counter for a few seconds, exerting pressure with your palm, to help break the cell walls for easier juice extraction.
- Warm grapefruit for an extra-sweet breakfast treat. Halve and section a grapefruit as usual. Heat each half for 45 to 60 seconds.
- Soften an underripe avocado (yes, avocados *are* fruit). Prick the skin and microwave for about 1 minute. Let cool before slicing.

◇   ◇   ◇

CRAN-APPLE SAUCE

◇ *Per serving*

119 calories
0.4 g. fat
(3% of calories)
3.6 g. dietary fiber
0 mg. cholesterol
4 mg. sodium

2 cups cranberries
2 apples, chopped

3 tablespoons maple syrup
2 tablespoons raisins

½ teaspoon ground cinnamon

*I*n a 2-quart saucepan, combine the cranberries, apples, maple syrup, and raisins. Simmer over medium heat, stirring frequently, until the berries and apples begin to soften, about 5 minutes. Use a potato masher to slightly crush the fruit.

Add the cinnamon and reduce the heat to low. Cook until the sauce is thick and bubbly, about 15 minutes.

Serves 4

FRAGRANT PEAR CHARLOTTE

3 pounds ripe pears, chopped
1 teaspoon grated orange rind
1 teaspoon vanilla extract
½ cup all-fruit raspberry preserves

¼ cup apple juice
12 slices whole-grain bread, crusts removed

2 cups nonfat vanilla yogurt
2 cups raspberries

*I*n a large frying pan over medium-low heat, combine the pears, orange rind, and vanilla. Simmer, stirring frequently, for about 30 minutes, or until the pears are very soft and thick. If necessary, drain any excess liquid.

In a 1-quart saucepan, combine the preserves and apple juice. Heat until melted and well combined.

Coat an 8½-inch round glass baking dish with nonstick spray. Place a round of waxed paper in the bottom of the dish.

Cut five slices of bread in half diagonally. Dip one side of each into the preserves. Fit the slices, dipped-side down, into the bottom of the dish, trimming the slices as necessary to cover the bottom.

Cut the remaining slices into 1-inch strips. Dip one side of each into the preserves. Fit the slices, dipped-side out, around the sides of the pan to completely cover.

Brush the bread with the remaining preserves.

Spoon the pear mixture into the pan. Bake at 450°F for 15 minutes. Reduce the oven temperature to 350°F and bake for 30 minutes.

Let cool in the pan. Cover and refrigerate overnight.

To serve, run the blade of a knife around the edge of the pan to loosen the bread. Invert the charlotte onto a serving plate. Peel off and discard the waxed paper. Serve the charlotte with the yogurt and raspberries.

Serves 8

Peach Soufflé

1½ cups chopped peaches
3 tablespoons honey

1 tablespoon lemon juice
½ teaspoon grated nutmeg

5 egg whites
⅛ teaspoon ground cinnamon

*I*n a food processor or a blender, puree the peaches.

In a 1-quart saucepan, combine the puree and honey. Cook over low heat, stirring often, for 20 minutes, or until thickened. Add the lemon juice and nutmeg. Cool the mixture to lukewarm.

In a large bowl, beat the whites until stiff peaks form. Gently whisk one-third of the whites into the peach mixture. Then fold the peach mixture into the remaining whites.

Spoon the mixture into an ungreased 1½-quart soufflé dish. Sprinkle with cinnamon.

Place the dish in a pan of hot water. Bake at 300°F for 1 hour, or until firm to the touch and browned. Do not open the oven door until near the end of the required baking time, or the soufflé may fall. Serve immediately.

Serves 6

◇   ◇   ◇

Marinated Figs and Apricots

8 ounces dried black figs
8 ounces dried apricots
½ cup orange juice
2 tablespoons lime juice

¼ teaspoon vanilla extract
1½ cups nonfat yogurt
1 tablespoon maple syrup

¼ teaspoon grated nutmeg
1 tablespoon grated lime rind

*R*emove and discard the stems from the figs.

In a 2-quart saucepan, combine the figs, apricots, orange juice, lime juice, and vanilla. Simmer gently for 7 minutes, or until the fruit is just beginning to plump. Remove from the heat, cover, and refrigerate overnight.

Spoon the yogurt into a cheesecloth-lined sieve. Place over a bowl and allow to drain until thick, about 2 hours.

Transfer to a small bowl. Stir in the maple syrup, nutmeg, and lime rind.

Serve the fruit with the yogurt mixture.

Serves 6

◇　　　　　　　　　　　◇　　　　　　　　　　　◇

TROPICAL COMPOTE

◇ *Per serving*

79 calories
0.4 g. fat
(5% of calories)
2.5 g. dietary fiber
0 mg. cholesterol
4 mg. sodium

2 star fruit	2 oranges,	2 tablespoons
1 papaya	sectioned	apple juice
1 mango	¼ cup lime	concentrate
1½ cups seedless	juice	
grapes		

*C*ut the star fruit crosswise into slices. Remove any seeds.

Peel and halve the papaya. Discard the seeds. Cut the flesh into thick slices.

Peel the mango. Use a serrated knife to cut the flesh from the large inner pit. Cut the flesh into thick slices.

Arrange the star fruit, papayas, mangoes, grapes, and oranges on a shallow heatproof platter. Sprinkle with the lime juice and apple juice concentrate.

Bake at 350° F for 15 to 20 minutes, or until all the fruit is warmed through. Serve warm.

Serves 8

NECTARINES WITH SAUCE CARDINALE

◇ *Per serving*

96 calories
0.8 g. fat
(8% of calories)
3.7 g. dietary fiber
0 mg. cholesterol
9 mg. sodium

1 cup raspberries
2 tablespoons all-fruit apricot preserves
1 teaspoon cornstarch
1 tablespoon water
4 cups sliced nectarines

*P*uree the raspberries in a blender or food processor. Transfer to a 1-quart saucepan. Add the preserves.

In a cup, dissolve the cornstarch in the water. Add to the saucepan. Cook over medium heat, stirring constantly, until the sauce is thickened. Cool.

Serve the sauce over the nectarines.

Serves 4

◇　　　　　◇　　　　　◇

APPLE TART

◇ *Per serving*

215 calories
1.8 g. fat
(8% of calories)
2.2 g. dietary fiber
1 mg. cholesterol
53 mg. sodium

CRUST
2 cups rolled oats
¼ cup apple juice concentrate
1 tablespoon ground cinnamon
FILLING
3 large apples, thickly sliced

½ cup apple juice concentrate
½ teaspoon almond extract
½ teaspoon ground cinnamon

1 envelope unflavored gelatin
2 tablespoons honey
2 cups nonfat yogurt
1 cup halved grapes

To make the crust: In a medium bowl, combine the oats, apple juice concentrate, and cinnamon. Press into a 9-inch pie plate. Bake at 350°F for 5 minutes.

To make the filling: In a 3-quart saucepan, combine the apples, ¼ cup of the apple juice concentrate, almond extract, and cinnamon. Simmer just until the apples are tender, about 10 minutes. Drain and let cool. In a 1-quart saucepan, place the remaining ¼ cup apple juice concentrate. Sprinkle with the gelatin. Let stand 5 minutes, or until the gelatin is softened. Cook over low heat until the gelatin dissolves. Remove from the heat and stir in the honey.

In a small bowl, whisk the yogurt until smooth. Add to the gelatin mixture. Pour into the crust and refrigerate for 1 hour.

Place the apples and grapes over the filling in a decorative pattern.

Serves 8

◇　　　　　　　　◇　　　　　　　　◇

SPICED APPLES

3 large apples, thinly sliced
1 tablespoon canola oil
½ cup cranberry juice
1½ tablespoons honey
¼ teaspoon ground cinnamon
⅛ teaspoon ground allspice
⅛ teaspoon grated nutmeg

*I*n a large nonstick frying pan over medium heat, sauté the apples in the oil until tender but not mushy, about 10 minutes. Remove and keep warm.

Add the juice, honey, cinnamon, allspice, and nutmeg to the pan. Cook over medium-high heat until syrupy, about 5 minutes. Add the apples and heat for 1 minute, turning to glaze the apples.

Serves 4

MICRO METHOD: Fruit Pies Made Easy

Fruit takes to the microwave like a duck to water. That's because microwaving is so fast it safeguards the luscious, just-picked flavor of vine-ripe fruit in a way no other cooking method can match. Here are some tips to keep in mind when preparing fruit pies.

■ To prevent boil-overs, be sure your glass or ceramic pie plate actually measures 9 inches across the top and is at least 1 ½ inches deep. (If your plate is smaller, reduce the amount of fruit filling or microwave the excess in custard cups.)

■ Microwaved fruit pies must be made in a prebaked shell. If the pastry is not baked first, it may absorb moisture from the filling and become soggy.

■ For best results, don't use a top crust.

■ A high, fluted rim on the pie shell will help contain bubbling.

■ Place a sheet of waxed paper on the bottom of the oven to catch any spills.

■ If the pie bubbles excessively, reduce the power to medium-high (70 percent) or medium (50 percent) and increase the time.

■ Microwaving time depends on the fruits used, with apples taking longer than most other selections. Berries cook very fast; check berry pies after 10 minutes.

■ When the filling is hot and has started to cook in the center, the fruit pie is done. As with all microwave recipes, the pie will continue cooking after removal from the oven.

■ You can microwave fruit cobblers and crumbles the same way as fruit pie fillings. However, be aware that the toppings will not brown.

The Shell Game

When it comes to the matter of a pie shell for your microwave pies, you can use your favorite recipe. But you have two choices as far as baking the crust goes.

You may prebake your shell in a *conventional oven* according to the usual directions: Prick the dough all over with a fork, then line the crust with a sheet of foil. Add some pie weights or dried beans reserved for this purpose. Bake the crust at 400° F for 15 minutes. Remove the foil and weights. Bake for another 5 to 7 minutes, or until the shell is lightly browned and thoroughly baked.

Or you may *microwave* it. Just be aware that although a microwaved shell can be quite tender and flaky, it will not brown. Here's how to microwave a crust.

1. Roll out the dough as usual and line your pie plate with it. Form a high, fluted edge to help guard against boil-overs.

2. Prick the crust with a fork at ⅛-inch intervals where bottom and sides meet and at ½-inch intervals over the remaining surface. That helps prevent shrinking.

3. Microwave the crust on full power for 4½ to 6½ minutes, or until the crust is dry and the bottom is opaque. (Rotate the dish after half the cooking time.) If you have a glass pie plate, you can also check through the bottom for doneness.

4. If your pie filling will be quite liquid, seal the prick holes by brushing the crust with a small amount of well-beaten egg yolk, egg white, or egg substitute. Microwave the crust on high for 30 seconds to set the egg.

◇   ◇   ◇

BERRY CUSTARD

◇ *Per serving*

102 calories
0.5 g. fat
(4% of calories)
2.3 g. dietary fiber
2 mg. cholesterol
77 mg. sodium

⅓ cup cornstarch
3 cups skim milk
⅓ cup honey
¼ cup egg
   substitute
1 teaspoon
   vanilla extract

2 cups sliced
   strawberries
1 cup
   raspberries

*I*n a 2-quart saucepan, combine the cornstarch with ½ cup milk until smooth. Whisk in the remaining milk and the honey. Cook over low heat, stirring constantly, until the mixture thickens to a syrupy consistency. Remove from the heat.

Place the egg substitute in a cup. Stir in several spoonfuls of the hot mixture. Whisk the mixture into the pan.

Cook over low heat, stirring constantly, until the mixture reaches a light-custard consistency. Stir in the vanilla.

Divide the mixture among six custard cups. Chill thoroughly.

Just before serving, top each serving with the strawberries and raspberries.

Serves 6

Stuffed Peaches

◇ *Per serving*

99 calories
0.4 g. fat
(4% of calories)
1.9 g. dietary fiber
1 mg. cholesterol
15 mg. sodium

4 large peaches
2 tablespoons lemon juice
¼ cup chopped raisins
1 tablespoon honey
1 teaspoon vanilla extract
1 teaspoon grated lemon rind
½ teaspoon ground cinnamon
⅓ cup low-fat yogurt

Scald the peaches in boiling water for 1 minute to loosen skins. Drain, slip off peels, cut the peaches in half, and discard the pits. Brush the fruit with the lemon juice to prevent discoloration.

With a grapefruit spoon or melon scoop, remove about half of the pulp from each peach, leaving a sturdy shell. Brush the insides of the shells with more lemon juice. Chop the pulp and set it aside.

In a small bowl, combine the raisins, honey, vanilla, lemon rind, and cinnamon. Add the reserved peach pulp. Fold in just enough yogurt to bind the stuffing together.

Divide the stuffing among the peach halves. Serve immediately.

Serves 4

Pineapple Fruit Cocktail

◇ *Per serving*

76 calories
0.7 g. fat
(8% of calories)
3.4 g. dietary fiber
0 mg. cholesterol
3 mg. sodium

1¼ cups chopped pineapple
2 oranges, sectioned
2 tangerines, sectioned
3 kiwifruit, sliced
2 tablespoons lime juice
1 tablespoon toasted coconut

In a large bowl, combine the pineapple, oranges, tangerines, and kiwis. Drizzle with the lime juice. Cover and allow to marinate in the refrigerator for about 1 hour.

Just before serving, sprinkle with the coconut.

Serves 6

FRESH TALK ABOUT FRUIT

Here's how to choose and store the cream of the crop.

Fruit	Look For	Storage
Apricots	Plump, juicy looking; smooth skin; bright golden orange color; yield to gentle pressure	Ripen at room temperature, refrigerate ripe apricots; will keep 3–5 days
Blackberries	Plump; bright color	Refrigerate, unwashed and uncovered; will keep 1–2 days
Blueberries	Firm; dry; well-rounded shape; bright purple-blue color with slightly frosted appearance	Refrigerate, unwashed and uncovered; will keep 1–2 days
Cherries	Firm; stems attached; good color	Refrigerate, unwashed and uncovered; will keep 1–2 days
Currants (fresh)	Firm; plum; bright red, almost translucent color	Refrigerate, unwashed and uncovered; will keep 1–3 days
Melons	Heavy for size; pleasant, fruity aroma; yield to slight pressure at blossom end	Ripen at room temperature; refrigerate ripe melons; will keep 2–3 days
Nectarines	Firm; plump; smooth skin; reddish yellow color; slight softening along seam edge	Ripen at room temperature; refrigerate ripe nectarines; will keep 3–5 days
Peaches	Firm; plump; slightly fuzzy skin; white to yellow to blush color; yield to gentle pressure	Ripen at toom temperature; refrigerate ripe peaches; will keep 3–5 days
Raspberries	Plump; bright color	Refrigerate, unwashed and uncovered; will keep 1–2 days
Rhubarb	Crisp, reddish green stalks	Refrigerate; will keep 3–5 days

Index

Note: Page references in *italic* indicate photographs.
Page references in **boldface** indicate tables.